HEALTH INEQUALITIES AND WELFARE RESOURCES

Continuity and change in Sweden

Edited by Johan Fritzell and Olle Lundberg

First published in Great Britain in 2007 by

The Policy Press
University of Bristol
Fourth Floor
Beacon House
Queen's Road
Bristol BS8 1QU
UK

Tel +44 (0)117 331 4054
Fax +44 (0)117 331 4093
e-mail tpp-info@bristol.ac.uk
www.policypress.org.uk

British Library Cataloguing in Publication Data
A catalogue record for this book is available from the British Library.

Library of Congress Cataloging-in-Publication Data
A catalog record for this book has been requested.

ISBN-10 1 86134 757 X paperback
ISBN-13 978 1 86134 757 2 paperback
ISBN-10 1 86134 758 8 hardcover
ISBN-13 978 1 86134 758 9 hardcover

Cover design by Qube Design Associates, Bristol.
Front cover: photograph supplied by kind permission of Getty Images.
Printed and bound in Great Britain by MPG Books, Bodmin.

Contents

List of tables and figures

Tables

Figures

Notes on contributors

Unless otherwise stated the authors are with the Centre for Health Equity Studies (CHESS), a multidisciplinary research institute jointly set up by Stockholm University and Karolinska Institutet, Stockholm.

Monica Åberg Yngwe has a PhD from the Department of Public Health Sciences, Karolinska Institutet. Her research mainly concerns the relationship between income and health, focusing on mechanisms of absolute and relative income. She is currently involved in a project further exploring relative deprivation and health. She is also a member of the project 'The Nordic experience: welfare states and public health'.

Johan Fritzell has a PhD, is a professor of sociology and affiliated research director at the Institute for Futures Studies. He has for many years conducted research on income and welfare inequality, and was a member of the Swedish Welfare Commission. He currently directs two larger research programmes on 'Welfare states, welfare services and welfare outcomes' and 'Segregation and its health consequences' and is co-director of a project about 'The Nordic experience: welfare states and public health', commissioned by the WHO Commission on Social Determinants of Health.

Örjan Hemström has a PhD in sociology and is an associate professor in sociology. He is currently involved in four research projects in the areas of gender differences in health and survival, alcohol epidemiology, socioeconomic health inequalities and occupational health.

Gunilla Krantz is a medical doctor by profession, and associate professor at Karolinska Institutet. She is at present working as senior lecturer in behavioural medicine at CHESS. She is involved in research on the division of labour, stress and men's and women's health in a Swedish context and on health outcomes of violence against women in intimate relationships.

Carin Lennartsson has a PhD in sociology and is a researcher at the Aging Research Center (ARC), Karolinska Institutet/Stockholm University. Her research mainly concerns intergenerational family transfers of both money and time across adult generations. She is also involved in research on health inequalities among older adults. She has been the project coordinator and responsible for the planning and conducting of the Swedish Panel Study of Living Conditions of the Oldest Old (SWEOLD) 2002 and 2004 at CHESS.

Olle Lundberg has a PhD in sociology and is Professor of Health Equity Studies. His research includes studies on welfare development, health inequalities, childhood conditions and adult health, income and health and sense of coherence. He is currently directing a project on the importance of relative deprivation and health, and is co-director of a project on 'The Nordic experience: welfare states and public health', commissioned by the WHO Commission on Social Determinants of Health.

Bitte Modin has a PhD in sociology. Her research concerns the short- and long-term health implications of childhood social disadvantage. She is also currently investigating the transmission of social disadvantage and ill health across four generations of children, parents, grandparents and great grandparents (based on the Uppsala Birth Cohort Multigenerational Study).

Viveca Östberg has a PhD in sociology and is Associate Professor of Sociology. She has published studies on the relevance of living conditions, for example family economy and social relations with parents and peers, for child health. Another area of interest has been children's welfare in general, where two important issues are how it can be described and how information can be collected. In line with this she has co-headed the data collection for the so-called Child–LNU and Child–ULF, in which representative samples of Swedish children aged 10-18 have been interviewed about their living conditions in a broad sense.

Eva Roos is a researcher at the Health Promotional Programme, Folkhälsan Research Center in Helsinki, Finland. She has a PhD in nutrition from the University of Helsinki. She has conducted research on inequalities in health and on social determinants of health behaviours. In 1998-2003 she coordinated, together with Professor Eero Lahelma, the Nordic project on 'Social variations in health – Nordic comparisons and changes over time'. She is currently doing research on social determinants of health behaviours.

Mikael Rostila has an MSc in sociology and is a doctoral candidate in sociology. He works as a research assistant on the research programme 'Welfare states, welfare services and welfare outcomes' located at CHESS. The subject of his dissertation is to study the links between different aspects of social capital and health both at the individual and the contextual level. In addition to this he has also published in the field of work environment and health. In 2006 he was a visiting scholar at the Department of Sociology, Harvard University.

Susanna Toivanen has a licentiate of philosophy in sociology, and is a doctoral candidate in sociology. Her research focuses on the association between adverse working conditions and ill health, and whether individual resources, such as income or sense of coherence, may influence this relationship. Presently she is investigating the effect of job control on stroke morbidity and mortality.

Acknowledgements

A book such as this is the result of the work and commitment of many people and institutions. Some of these people appear as authors, and we would like to thank them for their efforts and for their forbearance when we were lagging behind. In addition, a number of other people have contributed in various ways. We would like to express our gratitude to those who commented on our chapter typescripts at a two-day seminar in May 2005: Kirsten Avlund, Gunn Birkelund, Jon Ivar Elstad, Margareta Kristenson, Måns Rosén and Töres Theorell. Their comments and ideas were most useful and of the utmost importance to us.

The major part of the work on this book was carried out at the Centre for Health Equity Studies (CHESS), a research institute jointly founded by Stockholm University and Karolinska Institutet. We are grateful to our colleagues at CHESS for providing a stimulating and friendly work environment. We would also like to thank Carin Lennartsson for her invaluable contribution in the final phase of the work, to Bitte Modin for last minute comments, to Anna Bryngelson for assistance with data files, and to Mikael Rostila for helping us to organise seminars in connection with the work. Judith Black has, with her usual professional skills, helped us with language editing.

Much of the book uses data from the longitudinal Swedish Level-of-Living Surveys (LNU). We thank our present and former colleagues at the LNU project at the Swedish Institute for Social Research for their help in providing the data.

The writing of the book was facilitated by numerous research grants held by individual researchers. The main source of support, however, was a long-term research programme from the Swedish Council for Working Life and Social Research (FAS 2002-0840; 2005-1697).

Last, but not least, our gratitude goes to all the individuals who gave of their valuable time to answer the questions in the LNU. Without their contributions it would have been truly impossible to write this book.

Foreword

by Lisa Berkman, Professor of Public Policy, Harvard University

The Centre for Health Equity Studies (CHESS) has been on the leading frontier of research on the health impact of social and economic inequality. This book will become a landmark representing some of the most important work to emerge from this group to date. Over the last few years many scientists and policy makers have discussed the potential impact that social and economic policies may have on health. While the topic is clearly important, usually the results of analyses are disappointing. Here, however we have data from arguably one of the most forward-looking countries in the world informing us about the links between social and economic policies enacted during the period of growth of the Swedish welfare state and numerous health outcomes for a broad and diverse group of Swedes. A major economic recession during the 1990s provides us with further insight into the ways in which the welfare state policies enacted decades earlier may have softened the blow of the recession in Sweden. The book will have far-reaching effects.

Fritzell and Lundberg have assembled an impressive team of co-authors from CHESS to explore the full range of issues related to social determinants of health in the context of Swedish contemporary welfare policy. To understand the context of the study, it is helpful to understand that Sweden, along with a few other Nordic countries, adopted a welfare regime based on a social democratic model. Early in the book, the authors outline the unique dimensions of this model, quoting Esping-Anderson: 'Rather than tolerate a dualism between state and market, between working class and middle class, the social democrats pursued a welfare state that would promote an equality of the highest standards, not an equality of minimal needs as was pursued elsewhere' (Esping-Anderson, 1990, p 27). In comparison with the welfare models in the US for instance, Sweden exemplifies a broader, more generous, less exclusionary approach to welfare supports. The question then before us is 'Did this welfare state as constructed by the Swedes starting from the mid-twentieth century protect Swedish citizens in terms of the physical and mental health and functioning through the upturns and downturns of the economic cycles that occurred over the last 30 years?'. The policies enacted related largely to a commitment to full employment, active labour market policies, relatively generous benefit policies, high-quality public care services for children and older people and low poverty rates. How did economic and social conditions, demographic changes and state policy interact to impact on the health and well-being of Swedes?

As often is the case, the answer is complex but in this case very thoughtful. Fritzell and Lundberg and their co-authors address a number of health outcomes in the context of gender and life course issues related to social and economic inequalities integrating their findings in the historical period from the 1970s to 2000. Since the 1990s in Sweden brought a major recession, the analyses bring great insight into whether the policies were protective for the most vulnerable segments of the society likely to be impacted by the economic downturn. They explore the psychological and social pathways from sense of coherence and control to relative deprivation to see if these pathways might account for social variations in health. This book is concerned with understanding the consequences of social structures in terms of the resources and constraints they bring to individuals occupying such positions within the social structure. Fritzell and Lundberg are concerned with structures relating to occupational position, gender and age, immigration and social networks. An overarching theme of the book is that men and women of all ages will be better off as they have increasing command of resources. While the data address this issue in terms of the ways in which Swedish men and women are impacted, clearly the issue has broad implications for how all people respond to such circumstances. Many of the state policies the authors discuss directly increase resources whether they are material, social or psychological. They have not made what is often a false dichotomy between material and psychosocial resources, since both are related to health risks in the studies they present. The world is complex and this book does not attempt to oversimplify. Adding further to the complexity of the issues discussed here is the fact that economic and social inequalities in health are large in Sweden and other Nordic countries in spite of the welfare policies aimed to reduce blatant disparities. This challenges readers and authors alike to see current egalitarian welfare policies as an incomplete answer to social inequalities in health. Unregulated market forces may be expected to continue to impact on economic inequality and subsequently health inequalities.

A remarkable aspect of this book is the capacity of virtually all the authors to hold several themes simultaneously in each chapter – to be able to consistently explore the effects of economic inequality among Swedes of different ages, genders, occupations and marital – and immigrant and ethnic – statuses, often within the context of specific time period. Some of the findings suggest that immigrants have substantially higher risks for poor health outcomes, especially those from non-OECD countries, and only part of that risk is related to poorer economic conditions or low levels of social relationships. Clearly issues of social exclusion, a topic not discussed extensively will rise in importance in the coming decade. On a positive side, it does not appear that formal policies related to caring for older men and women reduces the informal social ties that also may play similar roles. Similarly, women, especially older women, in spite of Sweden's gender equality policies, unique in the world, suffer disproportionately in terms of income insecurity and functional outcomes in older ages. This is in part related to their marital status, age at marriage and labour history. Manual workers experience a range of risks in large part related to their current occupation. While earlier childhood experiences can be seen to set adults up for opportunities in adulthood, the evidence here suggests that it is these adult experiences which shape the odds of having major health problems in adulthood. The toll of accumulated experiences of economic hardship over the life course is also evident in these chapters.

The best part of this book is that there is no single 'bottom line' here. Many social experiences extract a toll on our health. Welfare policies, especially those that are consistent and in place during periods of economic hardship seem to be protective. Nonetheless, new social experiences emerge, with increasing waves of new immigrants, large increases in life expectancy beyond what we anticipated and new patterns of family formation. Such changes constantly challenge society to devise new ways to devise policies around work and evolving communities. These new experiences call for new policies – and so the story continues. But if you want to know how one very enlightened country with forward-looking policies and a deep commitment to collecting data on the health effects of such experiences has done over the last three decades, read on!

ONE

Health, inequalities, welfare and resources

Johan Fritzell and Olle Lundberg

Introduction

Health and inequalities are of great interest to most people. When asked to rank what is important in life the vast majority put health at the top of their list (Holmberg and Weibull, 2001). Health is also an everyday concern for most of us, and this is reflected in simple things like the reference to health in common greeting phrases ('How are you?') and when suggesting a toast ('Santé'). Inequalities, as in an unjust distribution of resources between individuals or groups, also seem to catch people's attention from an early age. The distribution and redistribution of resources is also the central aim of the political process. It is therefore no surprise that inequalities in health have generated a great deal of interest, among researchers, politicians and the general public alike.

Over recent decades research into health inequalities has produced a wealth of findings that have given rise to much debate. We would nevertheless argue that more remains to be said about the issue, both relating to the mechanisms that generate health inequalities and the policy implications these inequalities carry. In addition, we believe that there are insights to be gained by addressing these issues from a Swedish perspective. Sweden has been a special case in discussions about welfare states and welfare regimes, as an example of both success and failure. Sweden has also been referred to in the discussion about the size of health inequalities, and the possible links between health inequalities and social policies. In Sweden there is not only a strong tradition of research on health inequalities, but also a strong tradition of research into living conditions in general, often referred to as 'welfare research'.

In this volume we will therefore try to put health inequalities into the wider context of welfare resources based on the Swedish case; in doing so our work will rest on three different, but related, pillars. Our focus is to analyse, describe and understand health inequalities and how they are shaped, recreated, changed and influenced by social stratification, societal changes and public policy at the most general level. The field of health inequalities research has expanded considerably over the past 25 years or so and most of our questions and analyses are embedded in that field of research. Simultaneously we have another point of departure, namely the Scandinavian welfare research tradition. This tradition has long been studying health and health inequalities as part of the effort to understand how living conditions are structured and distributed. Since the present volume focuses on health in Sweden we also feel that it is appropriate to embed our findings in relation to the characteristics of the Swedish welfare state. Sweden is often characterised, in welfare state research, as the archetype of a particular type of welfare regime, according to the role played by the markets, the family and the state. The reason that we are interested in the configuration and activities of the welfare state in relation to health research is, of course, that the Swedish model is believed to foster equality.

One of the aims of this introductory chapter is to set the scene for the rest of the book. Starting with the context, that is, the Swedish welfare state, we will go on to discuss the definition and measurement of welfare in more detail. We will also discuss health inequalities and a number of key issues we feel it is important to highlight. Finally, the chapter includes an overview of the data to be used and a short presentation of the rest of the book, including some of the more specific research questions raised in the forthcoming chapters.

Swedish welfare state: distinct but changing

Since the by now classic typology developed by Esping-Andersen (1990), the practice of grouping countries into different types has become a whole industry in social policy research (Abrahamsson, 1999). The literature is, in other words, voluminous, as are suggestions about the basis on which classifications should be performed, the number of groups that might exist, which country belongs to which group, or the usefulness of a typology in the first place. In simple terms, Esping-Andersen's basic idea was that we could not understand welfare state development linearly. Welfare states have historically developed into systems with their own institutional logic, and the relative importance of family, market and state for people's welfare varies from one country to another. The concept of welfare regimes refers to precisely this, the various roles and importance of these three overarching institutions in the production of welfare (Esping-Andersen, 1999). Esping-Andersen identified three ideal types of welfare regime: the liberal, the corporatist/conservative and the social democratic model.

In this area of research, with heated and quite disparate views, there is hardly anyone who would question that Sweden is best characterised as belonging to the last of these three types. The social democratic model comprises a small group of countries, basically the Nordic ones, with a fairly distinct institutional pattern. In the words of Esping-Andersen:

> ... those countries in which the principles of universalism and decommodification of social rights were extended also to the new middle classes. We may call it the 'social democratic' regime-type

since, in these nations, social democracy was clearly the dominant force behind social reform. Rather than tolerate a dualism between state and market, between working class and middle class, the social democrats pursued a welfare state that would promote an equality of the highest standards, not an equality of minimal needs as was pursued elsewhere. (Esping–Andersen, 1990, p 27)

As stated above, welfare states are often delineated according to the balance between the family, the market and the state in terms of the importance, or the responsibility, for the welfare of individuals. In this sense the Nordic model is one that, to a higher degree than in continental Europe or the UK, the state has assumed responsibility for welfare. But how can the Nordic model be characterised more specifically? There exist no doubt several attempts to define the central elements of the Swedish, or Nordic, model (for an overview see Kautto et al, 1999). Without making any rank order, some central features of the model include: universalism, a commitment to full employment, active labour market policies, relatively generous benefit levels, high quality public care services for children and older people, high taxation, low poverty rates, and smaller inequalities, both between classes and genders. These features are a mixture of institutional principles, policy design and outcomes.

In the early 1990s Sweden was hit by an economic recession that, at the macro-level, had been impossible to foresee. In the space of just over a year, unemployment skyrocketed to around 10% (during the recession of the early 1980s unemployment never exceeded 3.5%). In three consecutive years the growth in gross domestic product (GDP) was negative, and the employment crisis ultimately hit all sectors and all socioeconomic and demographic groups. At the same time, Sweden received the largest influx of refugees in the postwar period, who encountered problems in finding work. Later on, crises in state finances following the economic crises forced politicians to implement cutbacks in almost all possible benefits and services and to raise all possible taxes. In short, these were turbulent years.

Did the recession that hit Sweden so badly (and Finland even worse) then lead to a systematic and qualitative change in the Scandinavian welfare state model? Such a question needs a qualified answer. On the whole, Nordic research into these issues has tended to suggest that this was not the case (Kuhnle, 2000; Kautto et al, 2001). The Swedish Welfare Commission carried out perhaps the most systematic analysis of the changes in Sweden caused by the recession (Palme et al, 2003). Their findings were also by and large in the same vein: despite the return of mass unemployment and the cutbacks in most social provisions, most of the general attributes of the Swedish model remained. They did, however, note the possibility of long-term consequences:

... it would be misleading to conclude that the model has been abandoned. Universal social services and benefits, as well as earnings-

related social insurance, still dominate the system. However, a number
of decisions, as well as non-decisions, might trigger more systematic
change in the longer run by changing the interest formation around
social policy institutions. (Palme et al, 2002, p 344)

One important implication of such a statement is, of course, that if the quality of
welfare state programmes, in cash and kind, is reduced, the upper and middle
classes will increasingly seek their own way of securing welfare. This in turn will
lessen their willingness to support public systems, which in turn will erode these
systems even further. Such a chain of consequences could obviously lead to
qualitative changes in the model in the future (Hinrichs and Kangas, 2003).

Yet another force is sometimes said to threaten the Nordic model, namely that
most often labelled 'globalisation'. It is, however, far from evident that globalisation
is especially threatening to the Nordic countries. Several researchers have recently
argued that, on the contrary, a country such as Sweden, with a long history of
free trade and experience of international competition, might be particularly
able to adapt to new circumstances.

Reform tendencies in Europe over the past 15 years have focused on issues
such as privatisation, more user charges and cuts and targeting in benefits; in
other words, tendencies that are the very opposite to the main characteristics of
the Nordic model. Most researchers note that the basic ideology of the welfare
state is resilient, that it is still possible to pursue Nordic social policies and that
they are possibly even especially beneficial in our times (Kildal and Kuhnle,
2005).

In this volume we focus on perhaps the most central aspect of welfare and
wellbeing, namely, health. We do this from the perspective of a country that has
been seen as the archetype of a type of welfare regime that is supposed to actively
influence people's living conditions and, in particular, the distribution of these
conditions. However, comparative work on inequalities in health has raised doubts
about the egalitarian impact of the Swedish welfare state in this respect (to be
discussed later on). The question is obviously open. In this book we will therefore
attempt to discuss how the actions, institutions and social programmes of the
welfare state are likely to have influenced the findings that we present.

Theory and measurement of welfare

Welfare is a concept with different meanings in different contexts; nevertheless it
essentially refers to a good, or at least decent, life. To wish people 'fare well' when
we part company is to wish them a safe journey home, but, in a more generalised
meaning, we are wishing them a good life. To fare well over the course of life is
therefore the essence of welfare, but there are nevertheless a number of meanings
attached to the concept. GDP is often presented and interpreted as a one-
dimensional, aggregate measure of welfare and prosperity. In welfare state research
and in the political debate, on the other hand, 'welfare' is used when referring to

certain aspects of social policies. Both economic growth and social programmes can be regarded as inputs of great importance for welfare developments but hardly as final measures in themselves. In contrast, the Scandinavian tradition of welfare research is concerned with the living conditions of individual citizens and their families. This tradition was initiated by the work of Sten Johansson and his colleagues with the 1968 Level-of-Living Survey (LNU).

Johansson (1970, p 25; authors' translation) defined level of living as "the command over resources in terms of money, possessions, knowledge, psychological and physical energy, social relations, security and so on by means of which the individual can control and consciously direct her conditions of life". Welfare, in turn, is defined as "... living conditions in the areas where citizens seek to influence through collective decisions and through commitments in institutional forms, ie through politics" (Johansson, 1970, p 138; authors' translation). This approach to welfare includes several ideas that strongly resemble earlier theoretical social policy writings, not least from the UK, as well as later writings in political philosophy and international social policy discussions. The central role assigned to *command over resources* was inspired in particular by the writings of Richard Titmuss (1958). Johansson's definition of welfare is closely linked to the commitments assumed by the welfare state vis-à-vis its citizens. This strongly reflects the writings of T.H. Marshall (1950) on the development of social citizenship rights in the 20th century.

There are, in fact, a number of important theoretical features seen in the definition and since we believe they are also essential to a proper understanding of the framework of this book, we list and discuss them here:

- the resource perspective that is explicitly actor-oriented;
- the good life, that is welfare, not directly defined;
- empirically a focus on negative conditions;
- welfare is a multidimensional concept and the dimensions are essentially non-comparable;
- collective resources are essential in many phases of the life course;
- the interrelation between welfare components, such as income and health, is fundamental.

In this definition the human being is seen as a conscious actor. An individual will, given the resources he or she commands and the context in which he or she operates, pursue whatever he or she regards as a good life. This is in stark contrast to much of the discussion about welfare that has need as the point of departure. This perspective is often, at least, based on the assumption that all people have the same needs and that these simply have to be fulfilled. In other words, if needs are universal and we are able to define them we have also defined the good life. This perspective leaves much less scope for individual action (for a detailed discussion of resources versus needs and need satisfaction, see Erikson and Uusitalo, 1987).

Second, the definition is indirect in the sense that the good life is not defined but rather left to the individual to decide according to his or her beliefs and preferences. Welfare resources, such as money, health or a good education, are essential in that they enlarge individual scope of action, but the decision about how to use the resources remains with the individual. Karl Popper, in our view, most forcefully elaborates the argument for such an indirect definition in his devastating critique of attempts to create the utopian good society. Popper (1969) claimed that utopian ideal conditions cannot be established without oppressing those who have a different view of what constitutes good society. Historically, there is good support for this argumentation, and Popper argued that we should rather aim for "the elimination of concrete evils" (p 361).

Third, and in accordance with Popper's view, Nordic welfare research has focused in particular on the opposite side of welfare, that is, on evil conditions or welfare problems. Of course, one cannot escape all normative elements in measurements, but it seems reasonable to assume that it is easier to agree about what constitutes misery or inferior living conditions rather than the opposite.

Fourth, this definition sees welfare as a multidimensional concept with essentially non-comparable dimensions. This diverges from welfare economics, which strives for a one-dimensional ultimate measure, and also clashes with the idea of seeing GDP as the ultimate welfare goal. On the other hand, it is very much in line with present discussions about and measurements of social inclusion in the European Union (Atkinson et al, 2002). It also coincides with Titmuss's view that welfare should be understood as a broad concept covering both the material and the intangible. Should we not, nevertheless, aim to be arriving at one single numeric welfare index? On the one hand, multidimensionality and incommensurability is quite easy to defend on strictly scientific grounds. There is no common yardstick by which we can compare, for example, income, health and social relations. How should we compare people who are wealthy but sick with others who are poor but healthy? Or, at national level, how should we compare 2% lower unemployment rates, or 2% fewer jobless households with a one-year increase of life expectancy? To do that we would have to find a way to rank outcomes in all different spheres of live along the same dimension. On a strict scientific ground this would be, to put it mildly, a difficult task. On the other hand, a single welfare index has a great appeal in itself, because it is easy to communicate. This is the great advantage of the United Nations (UN) Human Development Index, a composite index based on life expectancy, education and GDP, that was no doubt purposely constructed to combine non-comparable indices (see interview with Amartya Sen, *Finance and Development*, 2004). In short, a single numeric has great appeal but is still difficult to construct on a scientifically sound basis. The basic idea of multidimensionality may well lead to less apparent precision in our evaluation of social progress or regress, but in line with Sen, in his criticism of GDP, we should ask ourselves: "Why must we reject being vaguely right in favour of being precisely wrong?" (Sen, 1987, p 34).

Fifth, this definition focuses on "… collective matters that … arise from the demands and possibilities that all individuals face across the life-cycle" (Johansson, 1970, p 56; authors' translation). This implies that an evaluation of the level and development of welfare should focus not solely on individual resources (for example, health, income, education), but also on the availability and quality of collective resources. Welfare state institutions such as the healthcare system, the educational system and social insurance systems are an important element of such resources.

Sixth, and no less important, one should strive at analysing these various living conditions and resources in a comprehensive way. With a simplistic risk perspective you might fail to see how different forms of welfare problem are interrelated, whereas it is the welfare correlates that are central to the Scandinavian approach to welfare (Esping-Andersen, 2000). Analogously we believe that a proper understanding of how health inequalities are shaped cannot be achieved unless we study how different social determinants are interrelated in time and space.

The division of level of living into different components was inspired by the UN's work in the 1960s, and resulted in a list incorporating health, working conditions and economic resources, as well as issues such as family and social integration. The theoretical foundations of this level of living approach have much in common with the writings of Amartya Sen on welfare and wellbeing (see, for example, Sen, 1985a, 1985b). Sen has also referred to the Nordic LNU surveys as an important way of empirically examining diverse 'functionings' (see, for example, Sen, 1992, p 39). However, Sen makes a distinction between actual conditions, in terms of health, housing and so on (in Sen's terminology "achieved functionings") and the capability to function, that is, the means and freedom to achieve the conditions desired (called "capabilities"). In Sen's writings it is the capabilities that constitute resources, or the freedom to achieve functionings. Theoretically speaking there is much to support Sen's view on freedom. A common illustration of this difference is the comparison between two people, both of whom suffer from the same degree of under-nourishment or starvation. One of them is in this state because he is poor and cannot afford to eat, whereas the second has made a deliberate choice to fast. This aspect of freedom is not so easy to deal with in empirical research. In reality the domains included in the LNU are actually a mixture of living conditions ("functionings") and resources by means of which functionings can be achieved.

Measuring health status

There is a vast literature on the concept and measurement of health, and in this chapter we will only raise two issues of importance for the volume. First, we will study poor health and health problems rather than positive health. To focus on negative conditions is in line with the tradition of Scandinavian welfare research, but also, of course, in line with most research on health. Even though the negative concept of poor health predominates, concepts of positive health have also been put forward. The most famous of these is that already presented in the preamble to the Constitution of the World Health Organisation (WHO) in 1946: "Health is a state of complete physical, mental and social wellbeing and not merely the absence of disease and infirmity". This extremely broad concept of health is problematic, partly because of the immense problems in defining more exactly what a state of complete physical, mental and social wellbeing would be, and partly since it seems to imply that any deviation from this state is a health problem. The concept of positive health as defined by WHO is therefore more of an expression of a utopian ideal.

There are also scientific attempts to define and measure positive health. For example, Ryff and Singer argue that "… positive human health is best construed as a multidimensional dynamic process rather than a discrete end state. That is, human wellbeing is ultimately an issue of engagement in living, involving expression of a broad range of human potentialities: intellectual, social, emotional, and physical" (Ryff and Singer, 1998, p 2). Consequently, the Ryff scale of psychosocial wellbeing, argued to be a measure of positive health, includes dimensions such as self-acceptance, personal growth and purpose in life.

Although highly interesting from a strictly scientific point of view, it is apparent that a positive definition of health is not a good basis for policy; here the view of Popper (1969) that policies and interventions should aim for "the elimination of concrete evils" (p 361) rather than to achieve utopian ideal conditions is certainly applicable (see the earlier discussion). The negative concept of health, in contrast, cannot just be defined and measured in empirical research; it will also provide a better basis for policy and action. Since positive health is also proposed to be something different than absence of disease, it may not be caused in the same way as negative states of health (Blaxter, 2004). Positive and negative health, in other words, represent partly different dimensions.

The second question to address here is what kind of poor health we should measure. It is common to differentiate between poor health as (a) a medically defined disease; (b) an illness as perceived by a layperson; and (c) sickness disabling a person's functioning in the social environment (Blaxter, 2004). Although this typology may not be very helpful for the design of health measures, or for the choice between different measures, it indicates that poor health is not a one-dimensional entity. Rather, poor health includes both changes in bodily functions, the perception of symptoms caused by these changes, and their consequences for social functions. Therefore, it is appropriate that the measures of poor health that we employ reflect these different dimensions. Standard measures for examining population health, usually within the setting of population surveys, include both simple generic indicators as well as complex summary inventories (see, for example, Blaxter, 1989; Bowling, 1991, 1995).

The health measures we employ in this book are based on a mixture of the three aspects of ill health, with a focus on symptoms and functional consequences (for more details, see Chapter Two). Some of these are general measures (for example, self-rated health [SRH]), while others capture the more specific (such as musculoskeletal pain). By using several different outcomes we hope to give a more detailed picture of health as a welfare problem in Sweden.

In addition, to some extent we also present mortality data. Although death does not qualify as an indicator of health among the living, mortality calculations do give important information at group and population level. In most countries death records are reliable and valid, giving estimates of mortality, and thereby also reflect the 'true' mortality risks in a society. Mortality is therefore a major indicator of ill health and is used in all societies. A group suffering high premature mortality has a very extreme form of disadvantage. Therefore, mortality data are particularly useful in health equity studies. For example, class differences in mortality cannot be explained in terms of differential reporting, which is an inherent issue in studies using data on ill health.

In epidemiology, total mortality is often regarded as much too crude an indicator. In order to understand the aetiology there needs to be more analysis of cause-specific mortality. But there should also be an awareness that this introduces a number of measurement issues with regard to comparisons both across time and between social groups or nations. However, the main drawback with mortality data is that it does not adequately reflect the disease burden in the living population. In other words, there are health problems with low mortality risk that cause much pain and suffering at individual level as well as great costs in terms of sick leave, medication, medical treatment and care. Major examples are musculoskeletal diseases and most forms of reduced mental wellbeing. Consequently, mortality data, however important, cannot be relied on entirely in the context of the welfare perspective that is at the forefront in this book. Rather, we need a wide variety of data sources including aspects of health and illness.

Social stratification and health

Because this book is concerned with health inequalities (to which we will return later), it seems reasonable to also briefly clarify our perspective on social stratification. How the social structure affects individual life chances, that is, how a position in the social structure is linked to outcomes in terms of living conditions, including health and mortality, is one of the main issues of the sociological enterprise. All known societies produce inequalities and, like Grusky (2001), we can say that a stratification system is the system that produces inequality basically by two types of matching processes. On the one hand, there are social roles or positions that are related to unequal rewards, and on the other hand, there are individuals who are allocated to certain positions with certain rewards attached to them. A central indicator of this positioning in the social structure is often referred to as 'social class'. Division of labour and thus the occupational structure is often at the core of such discussions of social stratification. This structure, as well as the rewards attached to different positions therein, undoubtedly changes, but at a slow pace. This gave rise to Schumpeter's famous simile that the social structure is like a hotel, always occupied but by different people.

It is important to underline that there is no contradiction between this structural view and the view expressed earlier about the merits of using resources, the role of the individual and social action as a point of departure. They are in fact fully complementary. As Breen and Rottman put it (1995, pp 1-2):

> What emerges is a view of stratification as the study of social power and its distribution. By social power we refer to the resources that an individual possesses that enable him or her to undertake actions, and to the constraints attached to alternative choices of action. The actions of concern to us are those that affect people's life chances, the ability to share in the good things in life, both economic and social.

Although different perceptions and operational definitions of social class exist, the one elaborated by Erikson and Goldthorpe (1992) is nowadays the most commonly used in stratification research. According to them, a class schema should differentiate between positions within labour markets and production units according to the employment relation they typically represent. Empirically, such positions are based on occupational titles that are differentiated on the basis of ownership, supervision of others and level of qualification. This type of classification will be used in many of the forthcoming chapters, as will other measurements strongly linked to social stratification, such as income and its relation to health.

Health inequalities

Health problems – illnesses, ailments and premature death – can be viewed as utterly individual-level phenomena; individuals get sick, and individuals die. This view is reinforced by the fact that medical treatment is individual, and by the way in which behavioural factors such as exercise, nutrition, alcohol and tobacco are put to the forefront as important risk factors. Despite this there are clear and systematic differences in illness and mortality between social classes, educational groups, income strata, men and women, ethnic groups, regions and, not least, between countries (Macintyre, 1997; Marmot, 2004; Mackenbach, 2005a). This fact suggests that social structures and the processes that generate inequalities between positions in these structures are as important, or perhaps more important, than individual-level differences in inherited or acquired health risks. Poor health, consequently, is to a large extent a social problem and not merely an individual one, especially since individual behaviours are also socially determined to a large extent.

Yet, there has been some controversy over this issue. For example, Murray et al (1999) argue that the main inequality is between the ill and the healthy, or in their own words "... the variation in health status across individuals in a population" (Murray et al, 1999, p 537). The choice between a definition of health inequalities as inter-individual or inter-group disparities in health have both theoretical and measurement implications. When defining and analysing health inequalities in terms of differences in health between socially defined groups, we highlight the consequences of social structures in terms of the resources and constraints they bring to the individuals that occupy positions within these structures. In other words, we stress the commonalities in health risks that follow from certain social positions rather than the variability in health risks across all individuals in a society (see also Braveman et al, 2000). However, these two views are not mutually exclusive, and this volume will not only deal with health differentials between fundamental positions in the social structure (like social classes). We analyse a broad spectrum of social determinants of health, and while most of these are likely to contribute to health differentials between structurally rooted social groups, they may also contribute to health variations within such groups.

Health variation, inequality and inequity

Differences in health between groups are different in nature from differences in health between individuals. For one thing, genetic factors are likely to play a small and insignificant role for the production of systematic differences between social classes, since there is usually no reason to assume health-related differences in genetic set-up between those groups (Vågerö and Illsley, 1995; Davey Smith and Ebrahim, 2003). Similarly, differences in chance or bad luck can be ruled out. There are, however, systematic differences in living conditions, health-related behaviour and/or susceptibility to disease that ultimately lead to health differences between social groups. Health inequalities, as indicated by morbidity and mortality differences between social classes, educational groups or income strata, can be viewed as a very extreme form of inequality. Not only are people's positions in the social structure important for their daily living conditions, but also these positions systematically affect their morbidity and mortality risks, resulting in disproportionate levels of illness and premature death among those least well off. In this way the social structure of society quite literally affects people's life chances. Systematic health inequalities that are shaped by social arrangements can be said to be particularly serious with regard to injustice (Sen, 2002).

In the conceptual literature on health disparities the distinction is often made between health inequalities and inequities. Health inequity is closely related to injustice and is thus a normative concept. As Kawachi et al (2002) noted, we must then in principle make normative judgements in order to identify inequities – something that science alone cannot do. Having said that, and in line with what we have just said, we firmly believe that most of the inequalities between groups defined in relation to the existing social stratification systems in a society are also inequities. This is basically so since health risks, so-called social determinants, are unevenly distributed and closely related to a person's social position in the social structure. As Kawachi et al (2002, p 648) put it:

> ... most of the health inequalities across social groups (such as class
> and race) are unjust because they reflect an unfair distribution of the
> underlying social determinants of health (for example, access to
> educational opportunities, safe jobs, health care, and the social bases
> of self respect).

We could, accordingly, have used the term 'inequity' rather than 'inequality' in
the title to this volume. However, since what we are measuring is undoubtedly
health inequality, we decided to use inequality as our overall concept.

Health inequalities – now and then

Health inequalities have long been observed and commented on. For example,
in his famous work from 1845 *On the conditions of the working class in England*,
Friedrich Engels pointed to the damaging effects on health of crowded, poorly
ventilated and unclean dwellings, indigestible and unfit food, unsuitable clothing
and lack of proper medical care (Engels, 1969/1845, pp 127-34). Half a century
earlier, Thomas Malthus (1926/1798) noted that:

> ... it has been very generally remarked by those who have attended
> to bills of mortality, that of the number of children who die annually,
> much too great a proportion belongs to those, who may be supposed
> unable to give their offspring proper food and attention; exposed as
> they are occasionally to severe distress, and confined, perhaps, to
> unwholesome habitations and hard labour.

Some decades earlier still, the Swedish medical doctor Abraham Bäck concluded
that: "The poverty-stricken are ravaged by pestilence while few of the wealthier
fall ill" (Bäck, 1765, p 6), and he also pinpointed the reasons behind this: "When
I consider the causes behind diseases and excessive mortality among the peasantry,
and the worse-off in towns, the first and foremost are poverty, misery, lack of
bread, anxiety and despair" (1765, p 7; authors' translation). It may be noted from
these quotations that even early observers of the links between wealth and health
stressed not only the obvious consequences of absolute poverty, such as hunger
and lack of shelter, but also identified the importance of psychosocial mechanisms
such as "severe distress" and "anxiety and despair".

In more recent times, health inequalities, as measured by diverse socioeconomic
indicators, continue to be found (for example, Fox, 1989; Davey Smith, 2003).
There is no single country where health inequalities have not been found when
studied properly. Thus, health inequalities are universal, and concern not only
the worst off groups but cut across the whole social spectrum: the invariance 'the
higher the social position, the better the health' holds consistently true in a wide
variety of countries and for a wide variety of health indicators (Marmot, 2004).

What, then, do we know about the cross-national picture of health inequalities?

In the influential British Black Report (Townsend and Davidson, 1982) based on data from the 1970s, Norway and Sweden were singled out as having significantly smaller mortality inequalities than other countries. Although the empirical underpinning of this statement was not entirely convincing, later attempts to make direct comparisons between Sweden and Britain also led to a similar conclusion (Lundberg, 1986; Vågerö and Lundberg, 1989). More precisely, these studies showed that the size of relative inequalities, particularly for mortality, was larger in Britain than in Sweden, although the hierarchical socioeconomic pattern was fairly similar. An early comparative study of mortality differentials by education in the 1970s also found smaller relative differences in Nordic countries (Valkonen, 1989).

However, later and more comprehensive efforts to compare health inequalities were unable to reproduce these findings. Indeed, the general conclusion of a series of papers from the EU Working Group on Inequalities in Health was that inequalities in illness and mortality in the Nordic countries are as large as, or even larger than, other European nations (Mackenbach et al, 1997; Kunst et al, 1998). This was not only at odds with earlier results, but also challenged the view that the egalitarian welfare policies associated with Nordic countries would also reduce inequalities in health. A recent paper (Dahl et al, 2006) discusses at length the various mechanisms behind why we should expect the Nordic countries to produce less inequality, as well as a number of possible counterbalancing forces, which hypothetically could be relevant in explaining the evidence from comparative studies.

Part of the debate around international comparisons concerns issues of measurement, that is, how to conceptualise and measure inequality. Vågerö and Erikson (1997) noted that Mackenbach et al's conclusion is radically altered if, instead of looking at relative inequalities, we change perspective and scrutinise the absolute differences between social categories. When studying relative inequality, one reason for the seemingly unfavourable position of manual workers in Sweden seemed to be the very low mortality risk for non-manual workers. This issue has been discussed further in a number of review articles (Lundberg and Lahelma, 2001; Fritzell and Lundberg, 2005).

Another issue concerns the trends of health inequalities, both within nations and internationally. Without going into detail here, suffice to say that most of the recent international summaries indicate that health inequalities are not only substantial but also actually widening in many of the world's rich countries. This is, for example, the conclusion reached in a recent report by Mackenbach (2005a) for the UK presidency of the EU.

Understanding health inequalities: a life course perspective

Health inequality research has increasingly concluded that present health status is the product of social conditions accumulated over the entire life course, and even in part transmitted from one generation to another. This life course perspective is conceptually a theoretical model (for a recent epidemiological glossary, see Kuh et al, 2003), but at the same time it highlights the potential of studying changes over time either by means of reliable and comparable macro-data. We will also stress the emergence and continuation of health inequalities over time, or, in short, the life course perspective to health inequalities. We see at least five reasons for this. First, although different definitions on this perspective exist, it seems on the most general level plausible that health outcomes are partly the result of conditions both now and in the past. Epidemiological interest in the life course was recently strengthened by the idea of biological programming, which suggests that our conditions even before birth, in utero, are critical for adult disease risk (Barker, 1998). Alternatively, many have argued that it is rather the accumulation of conditions over the life course that determine present health (see, for example, Vågerö and Illsley, 1995). At any rate, one can expect a proper understanding of present health inequalities ideally to require knowledge of both past and present conditions.

The second reason for adopting a life course perspective in this book is that we deal with health inequalities as they appear in different phases of the life cycle, such as childhood, adulthood and so on. Thanks to our unique databases we have direct information not only for segments of the adult population but also for children and the very old, groups that are often neglected in studies of living conditions more generally. Third, in some of the chapters we employ a generational (birth cohort) perspective looking at health inequalities and, fourth, we have access to longitudinal micro-data that greatly enhance the possibilities to apply a life course perspective to inequalities in health.

Finally, particular interest in the life course perspective is warranted because one point of departure of our analyses is the discussion of the welfare state. Rowntree's (1901) classical poverty study among the working class in York noted that poverty risks varied across the life course. The expansion of institutions of the welfare state during the 20th century has, to a large extent, been motivated by a desire to equalise living conditions over the life course. Obviously this has had a great impact. Kangas and Palme (2000) have shown that the cycle of poverty has flattened out in many countries, not least the Nordic ones, indicating the importance of social policies.

Our data

The prime data source in most of the chapters is the *Swedish LNU* surveys, including some later extensions of that database that include children and the very old. The first LNU survey was conducted in 1968, based on face-to-face interviews with a representative sample of the Swedish population aged 15-75; the lower age bracket was later changed to 18. Follow-up surveys have since then been conducted at somewhat irregular intervals in 1974, 1981, 1991 and most recently in 2000 (a thorough description of the LNU can be found in, for example, Fritzell and Lundberg, 2000a; Jonsson and Mills, 2001). Guided by the theoretical base described above, the LNU aims generally to be a comprehensive database for analyses of the level of living of the Swedish population and inequalities therein. It includes questions about a number of spheres considered to be important for welfare. The survey has a panel design, but each survey also includes new younger generations and immigrants in order to remain cross-sectionally representative of the Swedish population. The analyses in this book will therefore be a mixture of truly longitudinal analyses and results coming from a repeated cross-sectional design in order to study changes over time at the more aggregate level.

The age span covered by the original series of surveys cannot give direct information about the conditions of the youngest and oldest population groups. To enable us to give an even more comprehensive picture of the welfare and living conditions of the whole population, two extensions were created more recently. The *Swedish Panel Study of Living Conditions of the Oldest Old* (SWEOLD) was initiated in 1992. It was based on interviews with all earlier participants in the LNU who were by then above the upper age limit. This survey was repeated 10 years later, incorporating again the new cohorts that had also passed beyond the upper age limit (for a detailed presentation of this study, see Lundberg and Thorslund, 1996a; Thorslund et al, 2004). Although the main bulk of this survey followed the earlier level of living studies, it also includes more questions of particular importance for older people, such as about functional abilities, and direct tests of physical and cognitive functionings among the oldest old.

A further extension was created to accompany the 2000 survey, namely a child survey, BARN-LNU. On this occasion, interviews were carried out with children aged 9-18 living in the same household as a respondent (for a detailed presentation of this study, see Jonsson and Östberg, 2001). Both these extensions will be used in our volume.

Research themes

In Chapter Two, Johan Fritzell, Carin Lennartsson and Olle Lundberg present an overview of the extent of and changes in health inequalities for various dimensions of ill health. The long perspective describes changes from the late 1960s to the new millennium with regard to age, class and gender inequalities as well inequalities related to country of birth.

Örjan Hemström, Gunilla Krantz and Eva Roos in Chapter Three look at how gender differences in health evolved over the period 1968-2000. They focus especially on how social factors contribute to gender differences in musculoskeletal pain and psychological distress. Risk factors include labour market participation, income, family situation and social network. Given that one of the most profound changes in most modern societies over the past 30 years is the increased labour market participation of women, it is naturally important to study the effects on health of this change.

Chapter Four by Johan Fritzell focuses on class inequalities from a generational perspective. Fundamental to the generational perspective is the idea that birth cohorts experience specific historical preconditions and circumstances. Nevertheless, the point of departure in this chapter is that the exposures of circumstances, that is, health risks, as well as vulnerability, are likely to be heavily influenced by position in the social structure. The life course perspective often stresses the importance of looking at time spent in different social positions, labelled the accumulation of risk (Ben-Shlomo and Kuh, 2002). It is these interrelations between generations, time and class differentials which are the focus of this chapter.

Working life is an arena that is known to produce health differentials between different social groups. Although physical working conditions are still hazardous for many workers, recent research into working life and health has focused on psychosocial working conditions. Yet health differentials are nevertheless to be found among people with similar working conditions. Antonovsky (1987a) put forward a salutogenic explanation to why some people remain healthy while experiencing adverse circumstances. According to Antonovsky, people may be better equipped to resist daily stressors and to stay in good health if they have a strong sense of coherence. The analyses in Chapter Five by Susanna Toivanen combine these two strands of research. As indicated by the chapter title, Toivanen analyses whether sense of coherence acts as a buffer against health hazards at the workplace.

An arena of similar importance for the younger sections of the population, as the working place is for adults, is in the focus in Chapter Six by Bitte Modin and Viveca Östberg. The demand-control-support model for studying working conditions among adults is here applied to pupils' situations at school. By using data representative of the Swedish child population and with direct information from children themselves, Modin and Östberg study how these conditions are associated with psychosomatic and psychological complaints.

The clear and systematic relation between income, income inequality and health has been a growing concern in recent health equity research, not least inspired by the work of Wilkinson (1996). In Chapter Seven by Monica Åberg Yngwe and Olle Lundberg, relative deprivation is addressed as a possible mechanism behind the income–health relationship on the individual level. The analyses review the literature and suggest two different ways of assessing relative deprivation empirically; first, through a membership group definition, and second, by self-rated deprivation (SRD) measured by specific consumption items. In both cases the analyses look at men and women separately and the clear gender differences in the effect of income on health, as well as the differences in the role played by relative deprivation, are discussed.

One theory about why income inequality could be related to population health status is that small inequalities foster trust, social relations and sense of belonging in a society, sometimes labelled 'social capital' (Kawachi et al, 1999a). The role of social capital is the focus of Chapter Eight by Mikael Rostila. He begins by discussing how this popular, but somewhat mysterious concept has been understood in the research literature (see, for example, Coleman, 1990; Putnam, 1993). The chapter demonstrates how the distribution of the preconditions for social capital, such as informal and formal social contacts, differ between various groups in Sweden and how this, in turn, influences health. Welfare state institutions have been seen as important for the emergence of social capital and for the development of trust and solidarity in society. The role of the welfare state in maintaining, creating, or perhaps even destroying the preconditions for social capital in a society is therefore also taken up in this chapter.

While children, adolescents and adults have been the focus of the preceding chapters, Chapter Nine is concerned with the oldest old. This group, which in numbers is the fastest-growing demographic category in most modern societies, is at the same time the most fragile with regard to health and functional abilities. It is thereby also an age group that is heavily influenced by the structure of and changes in the welfare state. Carin Lennartsson and Olle Lundberg examine, with data from SWEOLD, how gender inequalities in health are modified by marital status, and to what extent economic resources are important for the generation of such inequalities.

The aim of the final chapter by Johan Fritzell, Carin Lennartsson and Olle Lundberg is to discuss a number of pertinent issues in the current debate about health inequalities in the light of the findings of earlier chapters in the book.

Resources and the welfare state

As we noted earlier, one of the overarching questions in this volume concerns how our findings regarding micro-level relations between social determinants and health are influenced by the Swedish welfare state, in the broadest sense. We have here given a short presentation of the more specific research questions raised in each chapter. While these questions often deal with debates and inquiries within each specific field of research they are at the same time, albeit in different ways, related to the overarching questions. Consequently, Chapters Two, Three and Four all focus on changes over time in various forms of health inequalities. Chapter Two gives the broad picture, Chapter Three studies gender inequalities, while Chapter Four deals with social class differentials. These chapters cover the development of health and health inequalities in Sweden over more than three decades, including periods of welfare state expansion as well as periods characterised by welfare retrenchments. While these general descriptions of trends in inequalities do not address the possible impact of the welfare state directly, they form an important point of departure crucial for any discussion or analysis of that issue.

Welfare state institutions may influence population health and health inequalities in a number of ways. One way is to loosen up the links between social position and resources by increasing equality of opportunity, for example through good quality free education for all children. Schools are therefore central welfare state institutions, but as brought to the forefront in Chapter Six, the situation in schools and the way schoolwork is organised may also influence health among students. We hereby get an example of a more proximal and specific way in which welfare state actions and programmes are important for health.

An important set of welfare state institutions are the social insurance programmes, including, for example, old age pensions, sickness insurance and unemployment insurance. These systems, of a universal kind in Sweden, provide a 'latent resource' for all covered by the insurance, including those who are not presently ill, old or unemployed, and may therefore contribute to security and predictability more generally. More specifically, these programmes are important for individuals and families facing old age, poor health and unemployment since they alleviate the economic consequences of not working. As studied in Chapters Seven and Nine, this is in turn of vital importance for health, since lower income is closely linked to poorer health.

Welfare state institutions may also influence attitudes, behaviours and beliefs that in turn are of importance for health. One example of this is given in Chapter Five where physical and psychosocial working conditions are studied. Although a healthier working life has been the objective for a number of reforms, not least during the 1970s, adverse working conditions are still an important factor behind poor health and health inequalities. It is also studied whether sense of coherence, which is primarily an individual resource, modifies the health consequences of poor working conditions. Another example is found in Chapter Eight where the focus is on the prerequisites for social capital. Welfare state regimes have been used as a tool to try to understand cross-national differences in social capital, and central aspects of social capital like trust have been argued to be an important prerequisite for both welfare state actions as well as for health.

Finally, we would like to stress that the welfare state and its institutions are important only to the extent to which they provide its citizens with resources. These institutions, whether income maintenance programmes or social services, can be resources also for those who do not presently use them. Indeed, most people are better off when they do not make use of unemployment insurance or healthcare facilities, but having access to such good quality institutions adds resources to draw on for all citizens if the need arises. We will, in our concluding chapter, return to the concept of resources and how it can enhance our understanding of inequalities in health.

TWO

Health and inequalities in Sweden: long and short-term perspectives

Johan Fritzell, Carin Lennartsson and Olle Lundberg

Introduction

When looking at changes in health in Sweden during the past four decades it is important to bear in mind that a number of social and economic conditions have changed during the same period. The development of the Swedish (and Nordic) welfare state model has been summarised as "coming late – catching up" (Kangas and Palme, 2005), and this may also apply to the period after 1965. When the description starts in the late 1960s Sweden was not a country free from social injustice or social conflict – if indeed it ever was. In fact, the data we use – the Swedish Level-of-Living Surveys (LNU) – was in part the result of a discussion concerning the state of things in Sweden. When the Social Democrats launched their vision of a welfare state in the late 1920s under the label the 'people's home' (*folkhemmet*), it was declared that this would involve a "... decomposing of all social and economical barriers, that now divides citizens into privileged and neglected, into ruling and dependent, into rich and poor, propertied classes and impoverished, plunderers and the plundered" ("...*nedbrytandet av alla sociala och ekonomiska skrankor, som nu skilja medborgarna i priviligerade och tillbakasatta, i härskande och beroende, i rika och fattiga, besuttne och utarmade, plundrare och utplundrade*") (from a speech given in the Swedish Parliament in 1928 by Per Albin Hansson, MP, chairman of the Social Democratic Party and later Prime Minister).

Despite a number of large welfare reforms during the 1930s, and in particular during the postwar era, the 1960s was a period when 'uncomplaining poverty' was discussed. *The unfinished welfare* was an influential book (Inghe and Inghe, 1967) that described and discussed social problems such as poor housing and poor working conditions as well as groups that were excluded or left behind in the welfare development, including lone mothers, large families and low-income earners. Also a number of governmental committees were set up during this time to investigate social problems and to suggest reforms, including costs for dental care, medical drugs, pensions, unemployment benefits and family support.

Special attention was devoted to poverty and low-income earners, and a low-income committee was set up in 1965. As part of its work this committee financed the first LNU in 1968, in which around 6,000 people aged 15-75 were interviewed about their living conditions. When the results were published in 1970 and 1971 the reactions were often strong since it became evident that the living conditions of broad population groups were still far from the ideals of the 'people's home'. During the 1970s especially, and to some extent also during the 1980s, living conditions improved with rising incomes, shorter working hours, more involvement in social relations, and improved housing standards (Erikson and Åberg, 1987; Fritzell and Lundberg, 1994).

From the late 1960s to the early 1980s distribution of resources, especially regarding incomes, became more even. Typically, gender inequalities narrowed, not least with regard to labour market relations. The 1990s, on the other hand, became a decade characterised by economic crisis, mass unemployment and lower employment rates, increasing income inequalities as well as welfare state restructuring in a number of areas (Palme et al, 2003). The purpose of this chapter, then, is to analyse how health and health inequalities have developed in Sweden from the late 1960s to 2000.

Data, variables and methods

Our main data source is the LNU, which was conducted in five sweeps: 1968, 1974, 1981, 1991 and 2000. As discussed in Chapter One, the first survey was designed in relation to the multifaceted welfare concept developed by Sten Johansson. Hence, the interview included questions on childhood, family situation, educational qualifications, work and working conditions, economic resources, social relations, political resources, leisure time activities, as well as questions on health and healthcare utilisation.

In the first survey wave in 1968, a sample of approximately one per 1,000 in the ages 15-75 were interviewed by means of face-to-face interviews. In subsequent waves the people in the original sample were retained as long as they were 75 years old or younger, but additional samples of immigrants and young people were added in order to keep the cross-sectional nature of the survey. By keeping large parts of the studied subjects from one wave to another there is also a longitudinal component of this data, making analyses of individual-level change possible.

The main health measures are constructed from a long list of symptoms, signs of disease and manifest diseases, and are introduced by the question 'During the past 12 months, have you had any of the following illnesses or ailments?'. The items in the list include a wide variety of health problems such as coughing, vomiting, chest pain, gall bladder problems, nervous troubles, high blood pressure, diabetes and cancer. For each item the response alternatives are 'No', 'Yes, minor problems', and 'Yes, severe problems'. The list thereby comprises different kinds of health status information, including symptoms and feelings as experienced by the interviewee directly (like stomach pain or dizziness) as well as test results and diagnoses obtained from a physician (like anaemia or bronchitis).

Throughout this book most analyses will deal with two indices based on items from this scale, both of which will be introduced in this chapter. The indices are (a) *psychological distress* based on nervous troubles (anxiety, uneasiness or anguish), general tiredness, insomnia, depression/deep dejection, overexertion and mental illness, and (b) *musculoskeletal pain* based on items covering aches in shoulders, pain in back or hips, and pain in hands, elbows, legs or knees. These two indices are constructed as weighted sums of the values of the items included, where minor problems contribute with 1 point and severe problems with 3 points. The indices have been dichotomised, and a score of 3 or more counts as poor health.

In addition several analyses also use a measure of *mobility limitations* based on two questions on the ability to walk 100 metres and the ability to walk up and down stairs. Those unable to perform at least one of these are regarded as having mobility limitations. A third type of health measure frequently used throughout the book is *self-rated health* (SRH) based on a question that reads 'How is your health in general, is it good, poor or in-between?', with the two latter response alternatives making up the group with less than good health. Since the SRH question was introduced in the LNU 1991 it can only be employed for analyses of the more recent survey waves.

In this chapter we have also used the list of symptoms and diseases to capture the burden of ill health in total, and for this purpose we have used 42 items that were included in all survey waves from 1968 onwards. We calculate a summarised index with a theoretical range from 0 (no health problems) to 126 (severe problems on all items), but also an index of number of symptoms (0-42), as well as dichotomised measures capturing those free of health problems (score 0), and those with a heavy illness burden (score 6 or more).

The multivariate analyses in this chapter will make use of the repeated survey feature of the LNU. By collapsing data from 1968, 1981 and 2000 we will be able to analyse changes in general levels as well as changes in health inequalities over more than three decades. Apart from survey year, which will be included as an independent variable in order to capture changes over time, we will study health differentials in four structural dimensions covering central aspects of social stratification: *gender, age, country of birth* and *social class*. Although these sociodemographic groups are central they do not fully account for more specific and vulnerable groups, such as unemployed people, children, very old people, single mothers and people with disabilities. However, a selection of these approaches is used in other chapters in this book.

Gender

It is nowadays much more recognised both within science and politics that gender inequalities to a large extent are structural in nature, and in this sense, similar to class inequalities. Gender is thus a crucial aspect to take into consideration in the study of health and health development. However, when considering health differences between women and men this issue becomes somewhat more complex. In terms of mortality and life expectancy there seems to be a 'natural' difference, with women living somewhat longer than men. Therefore, although gender mortality differences vary both across societies and over time, thus implying that social determinants are important for this association (Hemström, 1998), an equal life expectancy could actually indicate harsh gender inequalities. At the same time women generally also report more ill health and disabilities than men of the same age, but the pattern is somewhat ambiguous and tends to vary with health outcomes.

To scrutinise gender differentials in health in Sweden and not least to focus on possible changes over time is all the more interesting since Sweden, and the Nordic countries, are most often regarded as being at the forefront of gender equality. Ever since Helga Hernes (1987) labelled the Nordic countries as potentially women-friendly societies, most welfare state researchers have noted that the Nordic countries stand out in terms of gender equality (for example, Kjeldstad, 2001; Gornick and Meyers, 2003). These observations are mostly based on social policy programmes facilitating women's autonomy in terms of various outcomes, such as labour market participation rates. How gender inequalities in health are affected by these and other features of Swedish society is less obvious. Gender differentials are therefore not only studied in this chapter, but will also be explored in more detail among adults (Chapter Three) and children (Chapter Six) as well as old adults (Chapter Nine).

Age

Age is often merely seen as a confounder, but even if health deterioration with increasing age is a biological necessity, the pace of this deterioration is very much a social phenomena. In many earlier studies we have highlighted the fact that general changes in living conditions are profound across age groups over time in Sweden, which of course, partly reflects cohort changes. While living conditions have improved considerably among older people over the past couple of decades, this is not true among younger segments of the Swedish population (Fritzell and Lundberg, 1993, 2000b). Therefore, age is also an important dimension to study in its own right. By using 10-year age groups we will give a general picture of health differences by age that roughly correspond also to the individual's place in the life cycle.

Country of birth

Nowadays more than one million out of nine million people living in Sweden were born in another country. Thus, although Sweden was previously known to have a very homogenous population, this is no longer the case. A key challenge for Sweden is to successfully integrate immigrants. Although international statistics on migrations are full of pitfalls and problems, we are able to say that in these respects Sweden today is a very heterogeneous society. For example, according to recent estimates the share of the population born abroad is lower in the US and the UK than it is in Sweden (Swedish Integration Board, 2003; OECD, 2005). The group of immigrants includes both labour force immigrants from Europe that moved to Sweden in the 1950s and 1960s and refugees from around the world that arrived later. Needless to say, there are differences within this group depending on their geographical, cultural and social origins, as well as the time spent in Sweden and the reason for migrating.

We will apply a fairly crude categorisation based on country of birth. Our sample size makes it impossible to do so according to specific countries of birth. But this is also a substantial matter, since it is unlikely that every nationality is facing different difficulties as immigrants in Sweden. One way to handle this is to group countries, according to the degree of economic development in their country of origin. This has proved to be important for labour market ties and incomes among Swedish immigrants (Edin and Åslund, 2001). The trichotomy we use in this book is people born in Sweden, people born in any of the 'old' member states of the Organisation for Economic Co-operation and Development (OECD) and people born elsewhere. There is, however, one important exception: people from Turkey are categorised into the third group.

Apart from economic motives the main reasons to immigrate to Sweden are political. With this admittedly crude categorisation we will, however, largely manage to capture both country of origin according to economic development and cause of migration according to economic versus political reason. Another feature of this crude categorisation of nationalities is that it will mask rather than highlight differences between groups. Consequently, any differences in health that we find between people born in Sweden, in OECD countries and outside the OECD are likely to be under-estimations of the actual differences by country of origin. However, were we not to find any difference between the three groups discerned we cannot exclude the possibility that some more specific immigrant groups are disadvantaged.

Social class

Social class is central for our analyses. Differences in resources and opportunities between social classes have existed throughout the 20th century, and the degree to which class inequalities in health remain is a central question of this chapter.

From the beginning of the 20th century a change in the class structure is notable both in Swedish society and elsewhere. The number of farmers and agricultural workers, together with unskilled manual workers, has declined. On the other hand, skilled manual jobs as well as non-manual positions have become more numerous. Together with this change in the relative size of social classes, the nature of classes themselves may also have changed (Breen and Rottman, 1995), that is, being a teacher or a clerk, for example, is different today compared to 50 or 100 years ago. Furthermore, changes may have occurred in the relation between class positions and welfare outcomes, in our case poor health and mortality, and these are the focus of this chapter.

The changes in class structure since the late 1960s also have a gender dimension. In the 1950s and 1960s many women were housewives and economically dependent on their husbands. The growing public sector that offered increased labour market opportunities for females changed the old attitudes about married women's employment, and in the late 1970s the housewife era came to an end (Axelsson, 1992). In 1990 Sweden had the highest rate of female labour force participation in the world with only 5% of women aged 20 to 65 being full-time unpaid homemakers (Nermo, 1999).

The social class measure used in this chapter and throughout the book follows the official Swedish socioeconomic (SEI) classification (Andersson et al, 1981), which has many similarities with the internationally well-known Erikson–Goldthorpe class schema (Erikson and Goldthorpe, 1992). The occupation of the interviewed subject is the base for the classification. The first distinction is made on basis of ownership, that is, between self-employed/farmers and employees. Within the group of employees classes are further defined by distinguishing non-manual from manual workers. Non-manual workers are divided into three classes according to the qualifications that typically are required in their occupation, namely, higher non-manual, middle non-manual and lower non-manual workers. In general higher non-manual workers have positions that require six years of education after compulsory school, and typical occupations include medical doctors, engineers and managers. Middle non-manual workers refer to occupations that require three to five years of education after compulsory school, and typical occupations are trained nurses and teachers. Lower non-manual workers have fewer years of education and many people within this class work as office clerks. Likewise, manual workers are divided into skilled and unskilled. Skilled manual workers include craftspeople, assistant nurses and so on, and unskilled manual workers include occupations such as cleaners and shop assistants.

Young adults with no labour market experience were assigned the class position of the father. Pensioners and housewives were assigned a class position according to their former main occupation, while housewives with no labour market experience were assigned the class position of their spouse. Respondents that could not be assigned a class were excluded from the analyses in this chapter.

The distribution over these four structural dimensions in our samples from 1968, 1981, 1991 and 2000 is shown in Table 2.1.

The main changes over time can be found for country of birth and social class. A clear increase in the share of the Swedish population born in another country occurred during the study period, and native Swedes decreased from nearly 96% to 87%. Our data also show, in line with official statistics, that the share of people living in Sweden born outside the OECD increased considerably between 1968 and 2000, indicating an increased ethnical heterogeneity of the Swedish population.

Table 2.1: Descriptive statistics of the structural dimensions included in the analysis (%)

Year	1968	1981	1991	2000
Gender				
Men	50.5	50.1	50.4	50.7
Women	49.5	49.9	49.6	49.3
Age group				
19-25	16.8	13.5	14.7	13.4
26-35	17.6	22.2	19.7	20.0
36-45	17.3	19.7	21.1	19.1
46-55	19.2	15.0	18.2	20.4
56-65	16.8	15.9	13.2	15.6
66-75	12.2	13.6	13.2	11.5
Country of birth				
Sweden	95.5	91.3	89.1	87.4
OECD countries	3.4	5.7	5.4	4.3
Outside OECD	1.1	3.0	5.5	8.3
Social class				
Higher non-manual	5.9	9.3	11.4	14.2
Intermediate non-manual	12.1	14.2	15.8	20.3
Lower non-manual	16.3	14.0	15.6	14.7
Skilled workers	16.7	17.4	18.2	17.6
Unskilled workers	34.8	32.1	29.7	24.2
Self-employed, farmers	14.2	12.9	9.2	9.1
n	5,488	5,215	5,169	5,142

As is apparent from Table 2.1, and also discussed earlier, the unskilled working class decreased in size between 1968 and 2000, while the group of middle and higher non-manual workers increased. The data presented here further indicate that the group of self-employed and farmers decreased from 1968 to 2000. This decrease can to a large extent be attributed to the shrinking agricultural population. In 2000 less than 1% of the working population are farmers.

Technically our analysis is performed by collapsing data from different survey years with the inclusion of year of survey (1968, 1981, 2000) as an independent variable together with our social differentiation indicators. The multivariate analyses will be performed by logistic regression. To test whether or not the patterns of ill health by each of these dimensions have changed we will include interaction terms between survey year and each stratification dimension in this chapter. In other words, in so far as such an interaction term is significant it implies a change of inequality according to the specific dimension (gender, age, country of birth, social class) in question.

Changes in life expectancy and mortality

Life and health are closely related to each other – without life it is not possible to speak about health or even welfare for that matter. As a consequence, mortality-based statistics such as infant mortality rates or life expectancy at birth are often used to describe public health, but also as general indicators of social development. For example, the 4th Millennium Development Goal adopted by the United Nations (UN) is to 'reduce by two thirds the mortality rate among children under five'. Moreover, the Human Development Index reported in the Human Development reports published by the UN Development Programme (UNDP) includes life expectancy at birth as one of its three components (UNDP, 2004). Even if life expectancy may be regarded as "... health defined in the simplest terms" (Blaxter, 2004, p 98), it reflects the fundamental issue of life or death. Questions regarding the level and distribution of health and welfare are only relevant for those alive. Moreover, the mortality figures underlying life expectancy calculations are reliable and cover the population as a whole.

Sweden has national mortality statistics dating back to 1751, and seen over 250 years the changes in life expectancy since the end of the 1960s are fairly modest. By looking more closely at this period, however, it becomes evident that the increase in life expectancy has continued up to the present time (Figure 2.1).

The life expectancy for new-borns has increased for both men and women, and in 2003 it reached almost 78 years for men and a little more than 82 for women. Although the increase has continued for the whole period the curve is flattening out for women during the last periods in the figure, whereas this is not the case among men. The gender gap in life expectancy has therefore decreased lately.

Figure 2.1: Remaining life expectancy for men and women at birth, at age 50 and at age 65

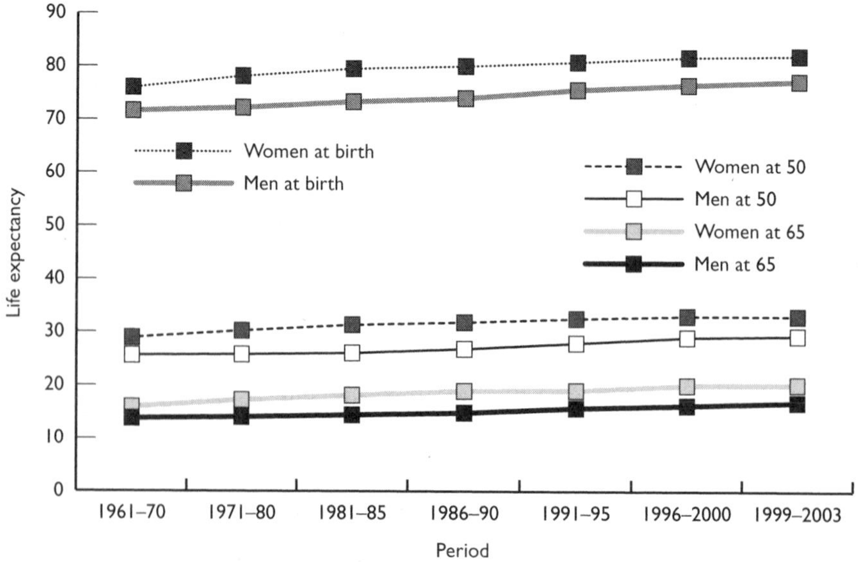

Source: Statistics Sweden (2005a)

Also in the higher ages there are clear increases in remaining life expectancy, in the figure represented by life expectancy at age 50 and 65 respectively (see also Chapter Nine). A man aged 50 has a life expectancy of almost 30 years in 2003, which correspond to an increase of more than four years since the 1960s. For a 50-year-old woman the corresponding increase is almost five years with a life expectancy in 2003 of a little less than 34 years. This increase mainly occurred before 1995, and since then female life expectancy from 50 and 65 years of age has remained stable. The stagnation of life expectancy among women in these ages are related to smoking habits, which has contributed to increasing lung cancer incidence among women during recent years, as well as an increase of alcohol-related mortality (NBHW, 2005a).

Apart from a tendency for life expectancy to stagnate among middle-aged and older women there have been substantial improvements in life expectancy for both men and women since the 1960s, and this development has continued also into recent times. In fact half of the improvement since 1970 among men has occurred after 1990, while for women it is about one third. The main reason behind this development is falling incidence as well as mortality rates of cardiovascular diseases, in particular myocardial infarction (NBHW, 2005a).

While the overall trends indicate substantial public health improvements in Sweden, there are still inequalities in mortality and life expectancy according to social class, education and income. Unfortunately the data available for analyses of trends in inequalities in mortality and life expectancy is scattered. Information on occupational social class for economically active people was collected in the censuses every fifth year, but since 1990 no new census has been carried out in Sweden. Through register information on educational attainment linked to mortality registers by personal identification numbers it is possible to follow mortality and life expectancy for different educational groups, but only from the mid-1980s (Statistics Sweden, 2004). Although based on a fairly crude division of education into pre-upper-secondary (low education), upper-secondary (intermediate) and post-upper-secondary (high education), these analyses reveal a clear pattern of inequality (Figure 2.2).

As for the population as a whole, life expectancy from age 30 has increased for all educational groups between 1986 and 2003. But it is also evident that there are clear differences in remaining life expectancy for 30-year-olds throughout the whole period, and that these differences are increasing, both relatively and absolutely. While the difference between high and low educated women was 2 years in 1986 it had become 4.3 years in 2003. In other words, the gap more than doubled (see also Chapter Four). Among men the corresponding difference increased from 3.4 to 4.9 years, which equals a 44% increase. Although none of the groups have experienced decreases in life expectancy, the sharp increase in absolute differences are disquieting signals of increasing inequalities.

The two figures also put a perspective on the gender differences in life expectancy. As can be seen by comparing the figures the male–female difference in life expectancy overshadows the educational differences; for most of the period

Figure 2.2: Life expectancy at age 30 by level of education: women and men

(a) Women

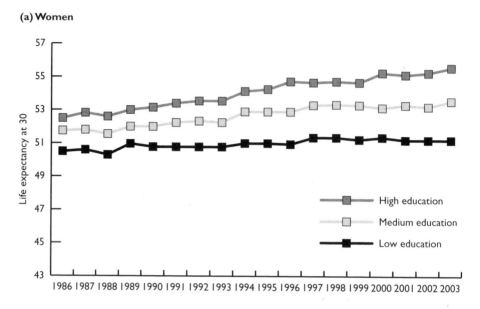

(b) Men

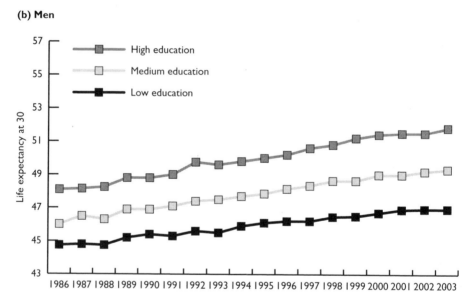

Source: Statistics Sweden (2004)

low educated women have longer life expectancy at age 30 compared with highly educated men. Only after the year 2000 highly educated men get ahead with a few months. This is largely due to poor development of life expectancy among women with low education; since 1986 life expectancy for this group only increased by 0.7 years. In fact, despite some jumps the main impression is that the curves are flattening out for all three categories of women during the second half of the period, while this is not the case among men.

In sum, the development of public health and health inequalities as described by changes in life expectancy is both positive and negative: both men and women live longer in general, but increases in life expectancy are graded by educational level. This means that life expectancy among women and those with only basic education have improved only modestly.

Health changes in Sweden 1968-2000

Although mortality represents the ultimate form of ill health there are certain drawbacks with mortality risks as a welfare indicator. Many diseases that cause pain, suffering, reduced functional ability and day-to-day problems are not fatal. In fact, increasing life expectancy in rich countries may imply that mortality is becoming a less reliable indicator of population health or changes of ill health among various social groups. Our purpose in this section is to give an overall picture of (a) long-term changes in the burden of ill health in Sweden; (b) how ill health is distributed across population groups; and (c) long-term changes of these population risks.

As described above, the main health question that we base our analyses on presents the interview subject with a variety of health problems, symptoms, signs of disease and manifest diseases. Since the 42 items we use hardly form a proper scale or index, we have chosen to present the data in different ways in order to get a fuller picture of the changes in the spectrum of ill health between 1968 and 2000. In Table 2.2 we present four different aspects of health derived from the symptom list, namely the mean number of symptoms, the mean symptom score (with minor problems contributing 1 point to the index and severe problems 3 points), the proportion having a symptom score of 6 or more, and finally the proportion symptom free.

The mean number of symptoms reported in 2000 is 4.9 among women and 3.4 among men. This is an increase since the late 1960s by about 0.5 symptoms. As usually found, men report less health problems than women. Basically the same picture emerges when we take differences in severity into account; the mean symptom score increases over time for both women and men, but the

Table 2.2: The burden of ill health: women and men aged 19-75 (1968, 1981 and 2000) (n = 15,799)

	Women			Men		
	1968	1981	2000	1968	1981	2000
Mean number of symptoms	4.5	4.3	4.9	2.9	3.1	3.4
Mean symptom score	7.2	6.9	7.8	4.5	4.7	5.2
Symptom score >5, %	44.0	41.6	48.2	26.8	29.8	32.7
Symptom free, %	14.0	15.0	10.3	22.6	19.0	16.0

score is consistently higher for women throughout the period. This increase in symptom scores is driven by a larger number of symptoms in general and not by a shift in the composition of mild and severe symptoms. In fact, the ratio of the symptom score and the number of symptoms remain stable throughout the period in both genders corresponding to a mean of 1.6 and 1.5 among women and men, respectively.

In line with this, the percentage of the population that have a symptom score of more than 5, for example by having 6 mild or 2 severe health problems, has also increased. Although this amount of symptom load is much more common among women, the increase over time seems somewhat stronger among men. The proportion of the population aged 19-75 that have not reported a single symptom during the past 12 months (out of the 42 symptoms included here) is, of course, fairly small. However, both among women and men there seems to be a clear trend towards a lower level, at least since the early 1980s.

These descriptions based on the list of symptoms are in a way imprecise since they mix more trivial health problems with serious diseases. However, in this sense it is also a good representation of the health profile of the population since it summarises all kind of health problems encountered by people in their everyday life. As can be seen in Table 2.2, a clear trend appears over the period; more symptoms are being reported, the symptom score becomes higher, the share of the population with a symptom score over 5 is increasing, and the share reporting no symptoms is decreasing. This raises at least two important questions; namely, if this development has been uniformly experienced across different sociodemographic groups, and how this trend can be interpreted in relation to mortality data.

The raw figures presented in Table 2.2 do not reveal to what extent the changes are affected by how men and women are distributed across, for example, social classes or age groups. Nor do the figures tell us to what extent risks of ill health have developed differently for people in different age groups, with different countries of origin or in different social classes. We now turn to these issues, by presenting estimates from logistic regressions. The estimates express the odds of having health problems for each category within each variable compared to a reference category set to 1. The survey year is also included as an independent variable in the analyses. At the bottom of each table we also show whether or not any of these differences have changed over time. If so, these changes are presented in graphs (calculated by multiplying main effects and interaction effects). The odds ratios (OR) for the survey year (1968-1981-2000) will tell us whether or not the risks for ill health have changed significantly over the time period once structural changes have been adjusted for, such as the ageing of population or the upgrading of the class structure. In so far as we can note changes thereof over the period, we will discuss them in connection with any such finding.

Analysing the odds of having a high symptom load (a score higher than 5) as an aspect of poor general health we find a stable development between 1968 and 1981, while there is a substantial increase by 2000 (Table 2.3). Across the whole

Table 2.3: Odds ratios (OR) for high symptom load (symptom index >5) by year, gender, age group, country of birth and social class

	OR	(95% CI)
Year		
1968	1.00	
1981	1.05	(0.97-1.15)
2000	1.38	(1.27-1.51)
Gender		
Men	1.00	
Women	1.92	(1.79-2.06)
Age group		
19-25	1.00	
26-35	1.16	(1.02-1.31)
36-45	1.32	(1.16-1.49)
46-55	1.77	(1.56-2.00)
56-65	2.67	(2.36-3.02)
66-75	3.38	(2.96-3.86)
Country of birth		
Sweden	1.00	
OECD countries	1.58	(1.34-1.85)
Outside OECD	1.49	(1.26-1.77)
Social class		
Higher non-manual	1.00	
Intermediate non-manual	1.08	(0.93-1.25)
Lower non-manual	1.42	(1.22-1.64)
Skilled workers	1.62	(1.40-1.87)
Unskilled workers	1.75	(1.53-2.00)
Self-employed, farmers	1.54	(1.32-1.79)
Interactions	*Significance*	
Year by gender	0.003	
Year by age group	0.000	
Year by country of birth	0.460	
Year by social classes	0.368	
n	15,495	

period, the odds of having a high symptom load is almost twice as high among women than among men. As indicated at the bottom of the table there has been a change over time in this difference (more technically the interaction term between year and gender is significant). Although statistically significant, there is no uniform trend in the relative difference between men and women – after a sharp decrease between 1968 and 1981 the gender difference has increased again in 2000.

Not surprisingly there are clear and systematic differences between the age groups in the odds of having a high symptom load. Health problems become

Figure 2.3: Changes in high symptom load by age groups: OR standardised by gender, country of birth and social class (average odds = 1.0, *n* = 15,495)

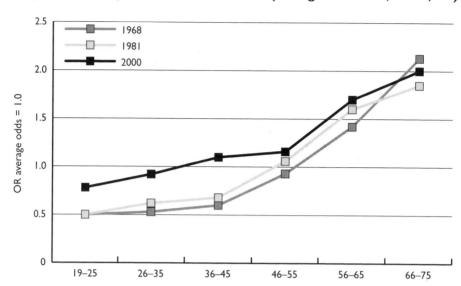

more common at higher ages, and this increase accelerates after the age of 55. However, these age differences have been changing over time, which has resulted in a different age pattern in 2000 as compared to earlier (Figure 2.3)[1].

The most striking differences can be found in the youngest age groups, where the odds of having a high symptom load have increased strongly over the period. This deterioration of health has occurred in all age groups included, with the exception of those aged 65 or older. The largest increase in poor health is found in the age groups 19-45. As a result, the age profile of having a high symptom load has changed over the studied period into a flatter one in 2000. Consequently, the OR of the oldest to the youngest has decreased from around 4.2 to 2.5 between 1968 and 2000.

Turning to the more specific indicators of ill health, Table 2.4 show the changes in prevalence of psychological distress, musculoskeletal pain and mobility limitations between 1968 and 2000. The health development according to the first two of these indicators is less positive compared to the mortality decline. The prevalence of psychological distress does decline between our first two

Table 2.4: The prevalence of ill health among women and men in the Swedish population aged 19-75 (1968, 1981 and 2000) (%)

	Women			Men		
	1968	1981	2000	1968	1981	2000
Psychological distress	19.9	16.8	22.6	10.7	7.9	13.1
Musculoskeletal pain	23.1	25.9	33.8	18.7	22.0	24.1
Mobility limitations	18.9	15.0	14.4	10.9	10.6	8.9

measurement points while it increases between 1981 and 2000. Thereby the prevalence is actually highest in 2000 for both women and men. For musculoskeletal pain we can observe an increase over the whole period. This negative development is seen for both women and men but the increase is much larger for women. Contrary to these changes, we find a decline in mobility limitations. This improvement appears to be more pronounced among women.

To reveal to what extent risks of ill health have developed differently for people in different stratification groups net of compositional changes logistic regressions

Table 2.5: Odds ratios (OR) for psychological distress, musculoskeletal pain and mobility limitations by year, gender, age group, country of birth and social class

	Psychological distress	Musculoskeletal pain	Mobility limitations
	OR (95% CI)	OR (95% CI)	OR (95% CI)
Year			
1968	1.00	1.00	1.00
1981	0.81 (0.72-0.91)	1.25 (1.14-1.37)	0.87 (0.77-0.98)
2000	1.29 (1.15-1.44)	1.74 (1.58-1.91)	0.82 (0.72-0.93)
Gender			
Men	1.00	1.00	1.00
Women	2.09 (1.90-2.30)	1.37 (1.27-1.48)	1.74 (1.56-1.93)
Age group			
19-25	1.00	1.00	1.00
26-35	1.05 (0.88-1.25)	1.63 (1.39-1.91)	1.27 (0.95-1.69)
36-45	1.20 (1.01-1.43)	2.11 (1.81-2.46)	2.02 (1.53-2.65)
46-55	1.46 (1.23-1.73)	2.91 (2.50-3.39)	4.15 (3.22-5.35)
56-65	1.82 (1.54-2.15)	3.75 (3.22-4.37)	9.12 (7.13-11.7)
66-75	1.88 (1.57-2.24)	3.69 (3.14-4.32)	16.45 (12.8-21.1)
Country of birth			
Sweden	1.00	1.00	1.00
OECD countries	1.84 (1.52-2.22)	1.63 (1.38-1.93)	1.57 (1.25-1.97)
Outside OECD	2.48 (2.04-3.01)	1.54 (1.28-1.84)	2.28 (1.78-2.92)
Social class			
Higher non-manual	1.00	1.00	1.00
Intermediate non-manual	1.21 (0.98-1.50)	1.24 (1.04-1.48)	1.35 (1.03-1.77)
Lower non-manual	1.38 (1.12-1.70)	1.63 (1.37-1.95)	1.88 (1.45-2.46)
Skilled workers	1.39 (1.13-1.71)	2.13 (1.80-2.52)	2.49 (1.93-3.21)
Unskilled workers	1.74 (1.44-2.10)	2.24 (1.92-2.63)	2.63 (2.07-3.35)
Self-employed, farmers	1.37 (1.10-1.71)	2.05 (1.72-2.45)	2.01 (1.54-2.62)
Interactions	**Significance**	**Significance**	**Significance**
Year by gender	0.177	0.004	0.012
Year by age groups	0.000	0.000	0.000
Year by country of birth	0.402	0.184	0.290
Year by social classes	0.570	0.097	0.099
n	15,487	15,492	15,507

are performed (Table 2.5). It can first be noted that all included variables are highly significant. In other words, the risks of having psychological distress, musculoskeletal pain and mobility limitations differ strongly depending on gender, age, country of birth and social class. Moreover, we see that for both psychological distress and musculoskeletal pain the odds are substantially higher in 2000 than in the beginning of the period. Controlling for changes in, for example, age and class distributions, the OR for psychological distress have increased with about 60% if we compare our estimates for 1981 and 2000, or 29% comparing the late 1960s with 2000. The corresponding increase over the whole period for musculoskeletal pain is 74%. For mobility limitations, on the other hand, we find a clear decrease in the odds, mainly occurring between 1968 and 1981.

Seen over the whole period the general social patterning of these indicators are otherwise strikingly similar. Women have significantly higher odds compared to men. The risks of ill health increase with age (but see further below). Furthermore, we find that immigrants have a much higher risk of ill health than native Swedes, and especially so among those born 'outside of the OECD'. Also, a typical class pattern is found, with ill health being much more prevalent among manual workers compared to non-manual workers.

However, as indicated by the significant interaction terms presented at the bottom of the table, some of these health differentials have changed over the period. The strongest and most consistent changes are found for age.

In Figure 2.4 a remarkable 'age equalisation' stands out. This equalisation is the outcome of a strongly negative development, with a sharp increase in the odds of having psychological distress among those aged 19-55 between 1981 and 2000. In fact, psychological distress is more or less equally common in all age groups at the turn of the century, except from a clear improvement in

Figure 2.4: Changes in psychological distress by age groups: OR standardised by gender, country of birth and social class (average odds = 1.0, n = 15,487)

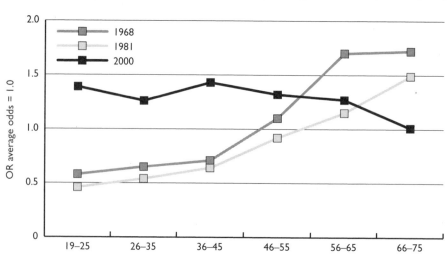

psychological distress in the oldest age group included. Thereby the OR of the oldest to the youngest has decreased from almost 3 to 0.7 between 1968 and 2000. The change is so dramatic that one may have doubts whether there is some data comparability problem at hand. However, the Swedish Welfare Commission reported on the basis of a different data material, and with a slightly different indicator, an almost identical development during the 1990s (Fritzell and Lundberg, 2000b; Palme et al, 2003). Moreover, as was presented earlier, our index of psychological distress consists of six items. When scrutinising our data we find that for all of them but mental illness the prevalence rates increase among the young (data not presented). This finding supports the conclusion that this change is real and not merely a change in the way 'anxiety' is used in everyday language.

The changes of the age pattern of musculoskeletal pain are less dramatic but still substantial (Figure 2.5). The risk of musculoskeletal pain has increased for all age groups included during the period, but the largest relative changes occur in the age groups 19-45. Unlike psychological distress there is still a clear age gradient in musculoskeletal pain, with the exception that pain becomes a little less common after the age of 65, that is, after retirement age.

Finally, the age gradient in the odds of having a mobility limitation has changed considerably since 1968. In absolute terms the most dramatic change is the strong decrease among the older age groups. Consequently, the OR of the oldest to the youngest has decreased from slightly more than 30 to 8 between 1968 and 2000. In relative terms we also find a rather strong negative development among the younger segments of the population. In many respects the change of the age profile is similar to the ones reported for the other indicators. However, the age gradient is much steeper for this indicator.

Figure 2.5: Changes in musculoskeletal pain by age groups: OR standardised by gender, country of birth and social class (average odds = 1.0, *n* = 15,492)

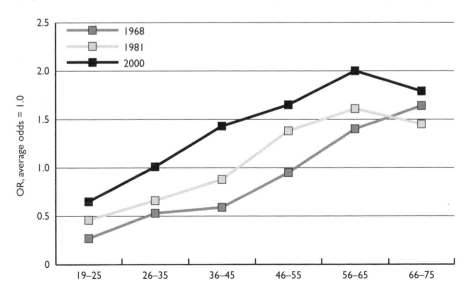

Figure 2.6: Changes in mobility limitations by age groups: OR standardised by gender, country of birth and social class (average odds = 1.0, *n* = 15,507)

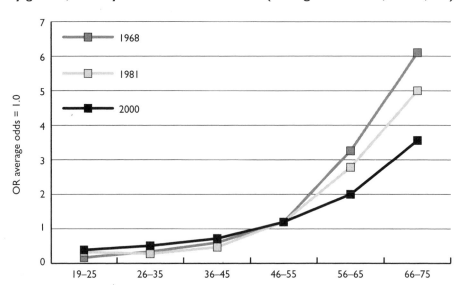

In sum, these dramatic changes of age differentials are likely, at least partly, to be understood as replacement of birth cohorts. The betterment of the health status for the oldest age group is in that sense rather expected. What is more intriguing and worrying is that, especially since the early 1980s, it seems that each new generation actually 'starts off' in a worse position than the generation before.

Although the gender profile seems to have changed in musculoskeletal pain and mobility limitations according to the statistically significant interaction term between year and gender, there is no clear trend detected between men and women. The result indicates that after a sharp decrease between 1968 and 1981, the gender difference has increased again in 2000.

Conclusively, there is no simple answer to the questions whether public health in Sweden has improved or deteriorated since 1968. Rather the picture depends on the selected health outcome – mortality risks have decreased considerably while psychological distress and musculoskeletal pain has increased quite dramatically. A substantial difference over the three decades studied is the change of the age profile that has occurred, partly through improved health at older ages (up to age 75) and partly through a negative development among younger age groups. This striking 'age equalisation' is therefore in part a public health concern of today, but also a potential public health problem of tomorrow.

Health changes in Sweden 1991-2000

So far we have looked at health development and inequalities in health over a period covering more than 30 years. We have done so by studying how different health outcomes vary between groups from the beginning of the period (1968), to the 'middle' of the period in 1981 and at the turn of the century (2000). However, the period 1981-2000 is rather heterogeneous, with political and economic changes that have to some degree reshaped Swedish society in fundamental ways. The economic boom of the late 1980s turned into the worst recession since the 1930s. The economic and labour market crisis that followed from this led to welfare state cutbacks that together resulted in a number of major changes in living conditions (Palme et al, 2003). In short, the 1990s was a period where the proportion of the population that encountered various kinds of disadvantage increased. Important features of this decade was higher unemployment rates and reduced employment, economical difficulties and an increase in health problems. Thus, the results showed by the Welfare Commission indicate that a closer look at the period 1991 to 2000 is warranted.

We have used two health outcomes to show the picture of health changes in the 1990s – psychological distress and SRH. The prevalence of psychological distress was around 20% in 1991, which is nearly the same as in 1981. In 2000 it had increased to over 30%. In the multivariate analysis we find an OR of 1.67 for 2000 compared to 1991, a change that is highly significant (Table 2.6). Consequently, the increased risk between 1981 and 2000 that was shown in Table 2.5 is in total attributable to changes during the 1990s. Further, the class differences in psychological distress are not very pronounced during this period, and the same could be said about the age differences. As was earlier described in Figure 2.5, there has been a strong negative development in psychological distress among the younger segments of the population that took place during the 1990s (not shown). As late as 1991 psychological distress was more common among older age groups but by the turn of the century it was almost equally common in all age groups with the least psychological distress reported by adults over the age of 65.

We also find a significant interaction term between year and country of birth, indicating that differences in psychological distress between Swedish residents born outside of the OECD and native Swedes has changed during the 1990s. The OR between residents born in Sweden and residents born outside the OECD was 3.7 in 1991 but decreased to 2.3 by the end of the century. This is mostly due to a more rapid increase in ill health among native born Swedes than among others, but the absolute level in reporting psychological distress is still much lower among those born in Sweden compared to other Swedes. Still, given the dramatic in-flux of refugees during the recession years, as mentioned in Chapter One, one would perhaps have expected increasing rather than decreasing differentials.

Also with regard to SRH we find deterioration of health for both men and women during the 1990s. For women the prevalence of less than good SRH increased from 24% to almost 30% between 1991 and 2000. Corresponding figures for men are 21% and 24%. However, from the logistic regression analysis we can conclude that the gender differences in SRH are modest, while there are sharp differences by age, country of birth and social class (Table 2.6). In line with

Table 2.6: Odds ratios (OR) for self-rated health (SRH) less than good and psychological distress by year (1991 and 2000), gender, age group, country of birth and social class

	SRH less than good	Psychological distress
	OR (95% CI)	OR (95% CI)
Year		
1991	1.00	1.00
2000	1.28 (1.16-1.41)	1.67 (1.49-1.87)
Gender		
Men	1.00	1.00
Women	1.17 (1.06-1.30)	1.85 (1.64-2.09)
Age group		
19-25	1.00	1.00
26-35	0.94 (0.77-1.15)	1.06 (0.86-1.30)
36-45	1.49 (1.23-1.80)	1.09 (0.88-1.33)
46-55	2.41 (2.00-2.90)	1.30 (1.06-1.59)
56-65	4.70 (3.90-5.68)	1.38 (1.12-1.71)
66-75	5.55 (4.59-6.73)	1.13 (0.90-1.42)
Country of birth		
Sweden	1.00	1.00
OECD countries	1.75 (1.43-2.14)	1.93 (1.54-2.41)
Outside OECD	2.49 (2.09-2.97)	2.67 (2.22-3.21)
Social class		
Higher non-manual	1.00	1.00
Intermediate non-manual	1.28 (1.05-1.57)	1.08 (0.87-1.35)
Lower non-manual	1.72 (1.40-2.11)	1.22 (0.98-1.54)
Skilled workers	2.25 (1.85-2.73)	1.17 (0.94-1.47)
Unskilled workers	2.75 (2.29-3.30)	1.58 (1.29-1.94)
Self-employed, farmers	1.78 (1.42-2.22)	0.94 (0.71-1.23)
Interactions	**Significance**	**Significance**
Year by gender	0.017	0.843
Year by age group	0.000	0.000
Year by country of birth	0.957	0.026
Year by social classes	0.796	0.784
n	10,177	10,153

earlier findings we also here found a marked increase in ill health among younger age groups (not shown). In the youngest age group included, the odds have increased by nearly 90% during the period and the increased gap is visible up to the ages over 46. After that age no obvious change in SRH is detected. According to our data both women and men report more ill health at the end of the period than in the beginning but the disparity between men and women is sustained during the period with women reporting more ill health than men.

Conclusion

The public health development in Sweden during the last three decades of the 20th century is not easily summarised, either in terms of levels of health or in terms of health inequalities. Life expectancy continues to improve, but the prevalence of psychological distress and musculoskeletal pain is increasing. Likewise, SRH shows a negative change over the past decade. This difference in results between mortality and morbidity risks reflects the different nature of various kind of health measures, and underscores the importance of including several aspects of health when assessing public health development. However, despite the fact that mortality and morbidity capture different aspects of the health spectrum they are related, and may well develop in the same direction. Our analyses also clearly suggest that the increase in health problems reported in surveys, and thereby the strongly diverging trends of life expectancy and health problems, is mainly a product of the turbulent 1990s. This is also reflected in a sharp increase in sickness absence that appeared in 1997 (NBHW, 2006). Apparently, whatever the causes are for the increase in illness and sickness, in terms of pain, psychological distress and sickness absence, they have not (yet) affected the major diseases that generate the bulk of mortality. However, looking more closely at the development of mortality the general positive trend is not shared by all groups. Rather, the improvement in life expectancy has been fairly bleak among the low educated, especially among low educated women. This development with improving life expectancy for all groups but increasing differences is interesting since it seems to parallel the development in Norway (Rognerud and Zahl, 2006).

How, then, should this development be interpreted? An often encountered problem in earlier studies of health inequalities, not least the Black Report, has been that a one-sided focus on *relative* differences between groups has obscured underlying improvements in survival and longevity among all groups. The problem, then, is that constant or even narrowing *absolute* differences transforms into increasing relative differences due to lower absolute levels of mortality, in other words because of smaller denominators. Here, on the other hand, we find increasing absolute differences, albeit all educational groups have experienced improvements in life expectancy.

This raises the question of how to understand and evaluate the development in terms of improving or deteriorating public health during periods of mixed trends. In line with, for example, Vågerö and Erikson (1997), we have previously argued that absolute differences, or even the absolute level of mortality among disadvantaged groups, are more suitable for evaluations of the public health situation (Fritzell and Lundberg, 2005). Accordingly, we believe that the weak development of life expectancy among those with low education, and especially among women, is a matter for concern.

According to the indicators of ill health analysed in this chapter, our main finding is that public health becomes poorer, and especially so during the 1990s.

One of the more dramatic changes is the strong increase in psychological distress that occurred during the 1990s. These results are supported by analyses of other data, showing that self-reported anxiety (one of the items in our index of psychological distress) has also increased considerably during the 1990s (Palme et al, 2003). This drastic increase in self-reported psychological problems of a milder kind evokes the issue of changes in reporting behaviour versus changes in health conditions. If the everyday use of words like 'anxiety' or 'nervousness' becomes more common or more accepted, the changes in psychological distress might not reflect a 'real' change, but a change in how they are reported. Although such changes in reporting are possible, we do not find it likely that they can explain the sharp increase in psychological distress during the 1990s. Furthermore we find an increase in all six items except mental illness. Hence, a reporting explanation must in such a case be relevant both for insomnia, depression and so on. Apart from the fact that drastic changes in the meaning or use of these words during a short period of time are not very likely, the predictive validity of the question on anxiety has also been shown to be good. Ringbäck Weitoft and Rosén (2005) found that not only is the simple question of anxiety related to strongly elevated risks for suicide attempts, psychiatric disease, all-cause mortality and hospitalisation in 5- and 10-year follow-ups, the relative risks are also stable over time.

Rather than being caused by a sudden change in reporting behaviours, we would suggest that changes in living conditions during the 1990s, perhaps in combination with changes in the predictability of life, has caused generally increased stress levels. For example, disposable incomes decreased in age groups under 50, as did the percentage with low incomes (Palme et al, 2003). An interpretation in terms of predictability is admittedly speculative, but consistent with the fact that the increases in psychological distress has been inversely related to age – if the future becomes more unpredictable it seems reasonable that this invokes more stress among younger groups.

Another health problem which has become more common is musculoskeletal pain, although in this case we find a steady increase throughout the whole period covered. It might be surprising that such disorders have become much more frequent in working ages, despite common assumptions that physical heavy work has become less frequent. However, the reduction of physically demanding work is much more modest than often assumed; in 2000 around one third of all employed had physically demanding jobs, and among working-class people two out of three had such jobs (Palme et al, 2003). Furthermore, recent research has shown that stress may also be a key factor here and work-related and other kinds of stress have been shown to be related to musculoskeletal pain (for example, Lundberg, 2002). In combination with increasing work stress (Fritzell and Lundberg, 2000b), not least in the public sector (Bäckman, 2001), this may have contributed to increasing levels of musculoskeletal pain.

While musculoskeletal pain has increased during the whole period since 1968, the ability to walk and climb stairs has in general improved during the same period. Although both of these findings are corroborated by other studies (NBHW, 2005a), they are nevertheless somewhat contradictory. How can increased pain from locomotive organs be combined with an increased ability to use them? Changes in levels of aspiration could explain increased levels of pain, but hardly the decrease in mobility limitations. However, if the increase in musculoskeletal pain is mainly driven by an increase of problems with neck and shoulders the findings would be coherent. This is also indeed the case; a separate analysis of the three items in the pain index reveals that the increase of pain in shoulders is much bigger than the increase for pain in back, legs and joints.

Although there are no clear trends in gender differences in health, we find some statistically significant changes. For musculoskeletal pain and mobility limitations the results indicate that gender differences decrease between 1968 and 1981, only to increase again in 2000. These changes in pattern might be a consequence of deteriorating working conditions in many female-dominated jobs in the public sector (see Chapter Three for a more detailed analysis of gender differences).

It is also important to stress that there are still clear and systematic differences in health according to social class and country of birth. We report health inequalities between people born in Sweden, in OECD countries and in non-OECD countries that are both substantial and clear, not least given the crude categorisation employed. It may be surprising to find that even the group born in 'old' OECD countries has elevated health risks. This may be explained by the fact that Finns constitute a large part of this group, as Finns (especially males) have high levels of ill health and mortality (Valkonen et al, 1992).

The remaining and stable class differences in health, both in relative and absolute terms, continue to pose a challenge for research and policy making alike. If these inequalities persist after more than 50 years of welfare policies, what, then, are the fundamental mechanisms generating class differences, and how can these mechanisms be altered? We return to these issues in Chapter Ten.

Note

[1] In order to be able to see not only how the respective odds ratios have changed relative to each other, but to what extent the odds for ill health have increased or decreased in absolute sense for each sub-group, the odds ratios presented in the Figures are deviations from the overall – geometric – mean.

THREE

Changing gender differences in musculoskeletal pain and psychological distress

Örjan Hemström, Gunilla Krantz and Eva Roos

Introduction

Changing gender differences in health in Sweden is an interesting field of study because gender equality has been prioritised, there is high labour force participation among both women and men, and there is a higher share of women in parliament than in most other OECD countries (Korpi, 2000). In a recent report on women's empowerment, Sweden ranked number 1 (overall score) out of 58 countries in gender gap ranking in the fields of economic participation, economic opportunity, political empowerment, educational attainment and health and wellbeing (Lopez-Claros and Zahidi, 2005). Nevertheless, many studies suggest that there are significant gender inequalities in Sweden in numerous areas, such as in the division of domestic responsibilities (Krantz et al, 2005), choice of educational career (Dryler, 1998), occupational opportunities (Nermo, 1999) and wages (le Grand, 1991; Thoursie, 1998; Bygren et al, 2004).

One issue that is of particular public health interest in present-day Sweden is trends in the development of common illnesses that account for the great majority of sickness absence and disability pensions, such as musculoskeletal pain and mental ill health (Lidwall et al, 2004). Gender differences in these common illnesses and sickness absence appear to have increased in the most recent period, possibly due to poor working conditions in predominantly female jobs in the public sector (Lidwall et al, 2004). The Work Environment Survey in Sweden observed that work-related illnesses in Sweden increased by two thirds for women and almost doubled for men between 1996 and 1998 (Statistics Sweden and Swedish Work Environment Authority, 2001).

Less is known about how gender differences in common measures of ill health have developed over a longer period. In this chapter we will analyse gender differences in health and social factors in the period covered by the Level-of-Living Survey (LNU) (1968-2000). Our aim is twofold: (a) to analyse whether there have been any changes in gender differences in musculoskeletal pain and psychological distress during 1968-2000; and (b) if so, whether there have also been changes in the social factors that contribute to gender differences in the two health outcomes. Of special interest was to investigate whether women's massive entry into the labour market has led to a narrowing or a widening of gender differences in musculoskeletal pain and psychological distress.

Background

Changes in welfare policy from a historical gender perspective

During the period covered by the LNU, living conditions changed more for women than for men. Women entered paid employment and the public arena in large numbers and women's economic dependence on their husbands declined greatly between 1968 and 2000 (Bygren et al, 2004). This development was driven by changes in Swedish welfare policies, particularly in the 1960s and 1970s. The 1970s has been called a decade of gender equality reforms, mainly with reference to women's increasing participation in gainful employment (Axelsson, 1992, p 28). Axelsson has described a large number of reforms that improved women's opportunities for earning a decent salary, such as the abolition of special 'women's wages' (1960), the expansion of public childcare (1965), individual taxation of work-related incomes (1971), parental leave benefits that include fathers (1974), and the legal right of parents of small children to work a six-hour day (1979). These changes affected women's lives more than men's, and men's participation in caring for small children is still modest. In 1997-99, one third of fathers still did not use any of their legal parental leave entitlement (Bygren and Duvander, 2004).

A previous analysis based on Swedish census data indicates that while women's participation in gainful employment increased from 54% in 1970 to 72% in 1980, mainly due to a massive increase in part-time work, the proportion of men in full-time employment declined from 85 to 80% (Hemström, 1999). Axelsson shows that, in the period 1968-81, the transition of married women from full-time homemakers to paid employees was common among all women born in the period 1920-49, but that it was greatest for those born in the 1940s (Axelsson, 1992, pp 33-6). By 1990, nearly as many women (78%) as men (80%) earned their own salary (Hemström, 2001a). However, in the 1990s, unemployment rose for both men and women although the most unfavourable development was observed for immigrants and single mothers (Palme et al, 2003).

Other important changes in social reforms and policies may also have influenced gender roles and relationships with possible consequences for health, for example lowering the retirement age (from 67 to 65 years), the liberalisation of the divorce legislation, and changes in the marriage subsidy (for OECD comparisons, see Korpi, 2000; Montanari, 2000; Ferrarini, 2003). The pattern of family formation and dissolution also changed in this period. Cohabitation (without marriage) has increased greatly in Sweden, as has the divorce rate (Bygren et al, 2004). Most social welfare benefits in Sweden are based on the principle of compensating for loss of work-related income, such as sickness absence, unemployment and parental leave benefits (Ferrarini, 2003). The structure of social welfare benefits, in particular parental leave benefits, is likely to have affected the timing of having children, and the length of time between the birth of each child, as well as general birth rates in the population.

There are probably historical changes in how men and women experience their social circumstances in a period. A number of changes from the 1960s onwards have clearly been driven by social welfare policies, such as the number of years of education and the ability to combine gainful employment and responsibility for small children. Also important from a health point of view are: the unemployment rate, the job structure and technological advances as well as the norms and attitudes of the period.

Gender differences in health

Analyses of gender differences in morbidity face a number of challenges, not least because of the considerable variation in gender differences across the different stages of the life course, as well as across general and specific morbidity outcomes (Macintyre et al, 1996; Arber and Thomas, 2001; Walters et al, 2002). Thus, empirical studies find relatively small gender differences in general health measures, such as global self-rated health (SRH), as indicated by samples from the Czech Republic (Hraba et al, 1996), Britain (Macintyre et al, 1996; Arber and Cooper, 1999), Canada (Denton et al, 2004) and Finland (Lahelma et al, 1999). In contrast, women across countries and age groups tend to report significantly more symptoms of mental ill health (Lundberg, 1990; Axelsson, 1992; Popay et al, 1993; Sweeting, 1995; Macintyre et al, 1996; Nazroo et al, 1998; Lahelma et al, 1999; Östberg, 2001a; Walters et al, 2002; Denton et al, 2004), although other studies find insignificant gender differences in mental health as measured by the General Health Questionnaire (GHQ-12) in a sample of two work organisations (Emslie et al, 1999, 2002). Musculoskeletal complaints such as neck-shoulder pain and low back pain are the most frequently reported symptoms resulting in sickness absence, followed by fatigue, headache, stomach complaints and sleeping problems (Statistics Sweden and Swedish Work Environment Authority, 2001). This is the case for both women and men, although in Sweden it is more pronounced for women and confirmed in studies from Norway (Brage et al, 1997) and the Netherlands (Bultmann et al, 2002).

Previous studies with an explanatory design demonstrate not only many similarities but also differences regarding the psychological and social factors that could cause gender differences in morbidity. Most studies tend to include the number of social roles (parent, partner, paid worker) and socioeconomic indicators, but some also analyse factors such as social networks and social support, work environment indicators, stressful events, domestic responsibilities and behaviours (Axelsson, 1992; Verbrugge, 1989; Lundberg, 1990; Nazroo et al, 1998; Lahelma et al, 1999, 2001; McDonough and Walters, 2001; Walters et al, 2002; Denton et al, 2004; Krantz et al, 2005) as well as one illness measure, such as long-standing illness or minor physical illness, contributing to other diseases or illnesses (Popay et al, 1993; Ringbäck Weitoft and Rosén, 2005).

The hypothesis of role enhancement versus that of double burden (see, for instance, Verbrugge, 1989; Hall, 1992) has been intensively discussed. Has entering the labour market been harmful or beneficial for women? Since the 1970s, much research has been devoted to gender differences in morbidity, but there are surprisingly few empirical analyses of changes in the gender differential in morbidity during periods of change in women's behaviour and their participation in the labour market. One Finnish study observed somewhat narrower gender differences in global health measures in 1994 than in 1986 (Lahelma et al, 1999). This was observed after a period of economic recession that was believed to have affected men's ill health more than women's.

There are three more general hypotheses regarding gender differences in morbidity. The first is gender differences in roles or exposure; the second is differential susceptibility to stress, psychosocial and physical exposure; and the third is gender differences in illness orientation. Some support at least can be found for the first hypothesis. Gender differences in morbidity tend to be smaller after social roles, socioeconomic and work-related factors and life stress indicators have been taken into consideration (Verbrugge, 1989; Lundberg, 1990; Lahelma et al, 1999, 2001; McDonough and Walters, 2001; Walters et al, 2002). However, there tend to be residual effects of gender that are not 'explained' by available psychosocial health determinants, and some of these effects are probably of biological origin (for example, Krieger, 2003).

Analyses of the second hypothesis are more inconclusive. Although there are many studies of specific determinants of men's versus women's health (that is, sex-specific analyses rather than determinants of the difference between men and women), these studies do not find a higher susceptibility among women than among men (for example, Fuhrer et al, 1999; McDonough and Walters, 2001; Walters et al, 2002). It is sometimes suggested that women's and men's health are related to somewhat different risk factors (Denton and Walters, 1999), but there are no overall assessments of whether such sex-specific associations also contribute to women's excess morbidity. Where men and women have been studied in social situations which are as similar as possible, which is difficult because of the gender segregation of paid and unpaid work, some studies have found similar associations between risk factors and mental ill health for both sexes (Emslie et al, 1999) while others report gender differences in effect of duration time in the job and musculoskeletal pain (Dahlberg et al, 2004). It is difficult to evaluate the susceptibility hypothesis because it is possible that biophysical as well as unmeasured psychosocial differences between men and women cause sex-specific effect estimates between an exposure and a specific outcome such as pain (Berkley, 1997).

A third psychosocial hypothesis concerns gender differences in illness orientation, that is, in making use of medical services and reporting ill health in surveys (for example, Hibbard and Pope, 1983; Verbrugge, 1989). It is difficult to establish a gold standard for 'objective morbidity' that could be used to test 'the reporting bias hypothesis'. The few such studies there are, not all of which have an objective standard, tend often not to produce the expected findings. Studies have reported that men are more likely than women to overrate common cold symptoms (Macintyre, 1993); older women have a greater number of functional disabilities that are not included in a global assessment of health (Arber and Cooper, 1999); and given the number and the severity of specific ill health symptoms reported, women did not rate their global health as poorer than men (Macintyre et al, 1999). This gives little support to the reporting-bias hypothesis. It should also be acknowledged that women visit doctors more often, not least because of pregnancy and childbearing, which might influence how women respond to and report their common illnesses.

Causes of gender differentials or similarities in morbidity are far from fully understood. It is not always the case that men enjoy better health than women, and there are probably changes in observed gender differences in ill health over time (Macintyre et al, 1996). There is little research into historical changes in health differences between men and women, and into the factors that might contribute to such changes, for example developments in social, economic and political factors (Arber and Thomas, 2001).

Analytical considerations

We will begin by considering the first two hypotheses identified above. To test the first hypothesis (gender differences in exposures) it is necessary to carry out an empirical study of gender *differences* in ill health and their determinants. Our main empirical analysis focuses on gender differences in exposure. To test the hypothesis that women or men are more susceptible, from the same level of stress or lack of health resistance resources, men and women must be studied in situations where occupational risks, own salaries, home duties and leisure activities are the same (that is, controlled for). This is very difficult and even samples from the same workplace find that there are gender differences not only in terms of home duties and leisure activities, but also regarding frequency and time spent in specific ergonomic work postures (Dahlberg et al, 2004). It is perhaps debatable whether we should see men's or women's greater susceptibility to a risk factor as due to physical differences between the sexes or social factors that lead to predominantly either men or women taking part in a specific activity, such as part-time working. Thus, if women are found to be more susceptible than men (to an exposure agent), this could still be due to gender differences in exposure.

Although we focus here on the determinants of gender differences in musculoskeletal pain and psychological distress (the first hypothesis), we will also look at the issue of sex differences in susceptibility (the second hypothesis) and gender differences in reporting ill health in surveys (the third hypothesis).

Research questions

It is as yet unclear whether life circumstances in which gender differences have narrowed have led to smaller gender differences in common illnesses since the 1960s. A large amount of research in this area has been devoted to the issue of whether paid work has been beneficial or detrimental to women's health. Even though work is health protective in terms of income and social support, job hazards and job stress are likely to cause work-related diseases (Hemström, 2001b).

The issue of whether women's increasing and men's decreasing presence in the labour market has been beneficial or not for women's and men's health over time is complex. It involves processes of selection as well as causation, and most likely such processes have changed between 1968 and 2000. If women are more likely then men to work part time and thus be exposed to work hazards for shorter periods than men, the balance between healthy and unhealthy aspects of work might be different for men and women. There are probably considerable changes over time as regards the type of jobs (and work exposures) available, the proportion of men and women working part time, and the degree to which specific job exposure is related to health outcomes.

We will analyse the relationship between ill health and level of labour force participation separately for men and women, first, because previous studies have found sex-specific associations between social, physical or other risk factors and general health (Denton and Walters, 1999) as well as pain (Berkley, 1997; Bingefors and Isacson, 2004; Dahlberg et al, 2004) and psychological distress (Roxburgh, 1996). Moreover, gender-specific selection into part-time working has been found in Sweden (Hemström, 1999). Thus, the more specific research questions are:

- Were there any significant changes in gender differences in psychological distress and musculoskeletal pain in the period 1968-2000?
- If so, are psychosocial, socioeconomic and work-related factors similarly important in contributing to gender differences in musculoskeletal pain and psychological distress in the period 1968-2000?
- Is exposure from paid work related to men's and women's musculoskeletal pain and psychological distress in a similar way throughout the period?

Material and methods

Study sample

Four cross-sectional samples of the LNU (1968, 1981, 1991 and 2000) were selected for the analyses. Age groups included in the survey vary from 15-76 (1968, 1981 and 1991) to 19-75 in 2000. We included those aged 20-64 (8,975 observations for men and 8,654 for women), as this corresponds to the time period for gainful employment for most people. Gender differences in health in younger and older age groups are found in Chapter Six and Nine of this volume respectively. In the 'explanatory' multivariate analyses, all observations with missing values in any of the included variables (1.8% of all observations) were excluded.

Variables

Dependent variables

We use two measures of self-reported ill health: musculoskeletal pain and psychological distress. The construction of these variables is described in more detail in Chapter Two.

Independent variables

Three variables of own labour market activities were included: paid work in the previous year (no paid work, part time, full time); own latest occupational position (unskilled manual work, skilled manual work, lower level non-manual workers, upper level non-manual workers [intermediate, higher-level non-manual workers and professionals], self-employed, unclassifiable); own gross income in the previous year (from registry) in quintile groups. For a full description of the Swedish socioeconomic classification (SEI), see Chapter Two. Paid work in the previous year was obtained through detailed questions about the number of hours spent in paid employment, self-employment or assisting a self-employed member of the family. Hours of paid work were aggregated to annual figures, and those who were in paid work for at least 1,800 hours (34.6 hours per week) were classified as full-time workers.

We were particularly interested in the changes in men's and women's own resources and social status in society in the period 1968-2000, and we do not therefore follow the common practice of using household income or information about a spouse's occupation for women (or occasionally men) not in the labour market. The income measure, presented in quintiles based on the total sample in each period, is an attempt to assign a relative individual income position for both sexes in each period. In 1968, more than 20% of the women (aged 20-64) had no own gross income. There is no adjustment for inflation because the income measure is an indicator of relative position in the income hierarchy, something that has been suggested to be especially important for health (Wilkinson, 1996).

The variables for family and social relations are: living alone (yes/no), marital status (never married, married, divorced, widowed), number of children in the home (none, one, two, three or more) and a variable for social network. We constructed an additive index of social contacts based on four questions about how often friends and relatives visited the respondent and how often the respondent visited them. 'No contacts' was given the value 0, 'seldom' was given the value 1, and 'often' 2. The range of the index (0-8) was skewed towards frequent social contacts with a mean of 5.18. We also observed a clear statistical shift in the proportion of those scoring 3 on the index (4.5%) as compared to those scoring 4 (34.8%). Accordingly, respondents with less than 4 on the index were regarded as having a low level of social network, 4–5 as medium, and 6 or higher as a high level of social network.

A question about 'running a household' in the previous year is regarded as an indicator of responsibility for the household (yes, no). Unfortunately, unlike paid work, this variable could not be classified as part-time or full-time involvement in household (unpaid) work.

We selected four work environment factors in 1981 and 2000: *ergonomic load* (an index of heavy lifting, unsuitable work postures, daily perspiring from work, physically demanding work tasks, physical exhaustion and repetitive movements); *chemical/physical exposure* (an index of exposure to dirt, noise, gas/dust/smoke and poison/acid/explosive substances); *psychological demands* (an index of hectic work, mental exhaustion and mental efforts); and *varied work*. Varied work (yes/no) is an indicator of skill discretion that is one component of decision latitude in the demand–control model (Karasek, 1979; Karasek and Theorell, 1990; see also Chapters Five and Six). Because questions of decision authority are not relevant to self-employed people we could not include such items in the analyses. The three indexes were constructed in a similar way, and split into low, medium and high exposure levels. 'Low' means exposure to none of six ergonomic items, none of four chemical/physical items, and none of three items of psychological demands. 'Medium' exposure means one to three 'yes' answers to ergonomic items, one or two to chemical/physical items and one to psychological demands. 'High' exposure is classified as at least four yes answers to ergonomic loads, at least three to chemical/physical substances and at least two to psychological demands. All work environment factors include the category 'not in paid work'.

The correlations between psychological distress and musculoskeletal pain were not very high, although found to be higher for women (0.27 to 0.32) than for men (0.19 to 0.24) throughout the study period. This indicates that co-morbidity between musculoskeletal pain and psychological distress is more common among women than among men. Therefore we use musculoskeletal pain as a contributing factor to psychological distress and vice versa.

Statistical methods

The data is described by, first, calculating the prevalence of ill health as rate differences between women and men, and relative health differences for women compared with men across the entire period. The pattern of ill health in different age groups for men and women is shown in Figure 3.1.

Analyses of changes in all independent variables in the period were performed for men and women. In order to estimate the rate of change regarding the concentration of women and men into various groups, we used the proportion of women in each category. The chi-square test was applied in these analyses.

By means of multivariate logistic regression modelling, we estimated relative gender differences in each observation year, using men as the reference category and controlling for age in the first model. Next, we estimated one independent variable at a time into the regression to be able to evaluate each variable's contribution to the initial age-adjusted gender difference. Changes over time in the contribution of various factors to gender differences in musculoskeletal pain and psychological distress are of particular interest.

Possible sex-specific relationships between paid work factors and ill health were analysed separately for men and women using logistic regressions and adjusting for age.

Results

Changes in health

Women reported significantly more musculoskeletal pain and psychological distress than men in all observation years (Table 3.1). These differences widened for musculoskeletal pain after 1981, both in relative and absolute terms. In 2000, the gender difference in musculoskeletal pain had more than doubled compared to 1968. Gender differences in psychological distress varied somewhat over time, but we could not observe any clear direction of change for this outcome. These findings suggest that musculoskeletal pain accounted for most of the changes in health differentials between men and women in the period 1981-2000.

Table 3.1: Changing health differentials between men and women, 1968-2000, expressed as prevalence differences (women's prevalence-men's prevalence) and as relative differences (age-adjusted odds ratios [OR] in logistic regressions)

	1968	1981	1991	2000
Musculoskeletal pain				
Prevalence among women[a]	20.5	24.3	28.7	31.8
Prevalence among men[a]	17.5	21.7	22.7	23.7
Difference women–men	3.0	2.6	6.0	8.1
Age-adjusted OR	1.24	1.16	1.38	1.54
(women relative to men and 95% CI)	(1.07-1.44)	(1.01-1.34)	(1.20-1.59)	(1.35-1.76)
n	4,598	4,315	4,290	4,383
Psychological distress				
Prevalence among women[a]	18.1	15.3	14.5	23.4
Prevalence among men[a]	10.1	7.4	8.7	13.4
Difference women–men	8.0	7.9	5.8	10.0
Age-adjusted OR	2.00	2.27	1.79	1.97
(women relative to men and 95% CI)	(1.68-2.38)	(1.86-2.77)	(1.48-2.18)	(1.68-2.31)
n	4,598	4,315	4,286	4,374

Note: [a] Age standardised by the direct method and five-year age groups. The age distribution in the entire sample for all periods was used as the reference population.

The prevalence of pain did not increase in the same way for all age groups of men and women from 1968 to 2000 (Figure 3.1(a)). The increase was particularly pronounced for women aged 40-59, while it was modest for men in the same age group.

Psychological distress demonstrates a different pattern. In 1968, 60- to 64-year olds had the highest prevalence. This was not the case in 2000 due to a large increase of psychological distress among young adults between 1991 and 2000 (Figure 3.1(b)).

When changes in male and female prevalence of musculoskeletal pain and psychological distress are presented as absolute gender differences, it is evident that gender differences in musculoskeletal pain have changed in an age-specific way. After 1981, the increasing gender differences in pain are most evident in those aged 40-59 (Figure 3.1(c)). Gender differences in psychological distress have changed in a similar way across the age groups (Figure 3.1(d)).

Changes in social factors

For both men and women, significant changes in the distribution were observed for all social and economic factors in the period 1968 to 2000 (not shown in a table). The proportion of married people in the population fell, divorce rates rose, and consequently more people were living alone. The number of children in the home declined for both men and women. On the other hand, social networks improved.

Women's income levels significantly approached those of men but failed to reach comparable levels. The proportion of men in the lowest income quintile increased even as it decreased for women. Nevertheless, in 2000 only 10% of the women were in the highest quintile as opposed to 29% of the men.

When one looks at socioeconomic groups, the gap between men and women also levelled out, with the proportion of women who were skilled workers and upper non-manual workers increasing but not reaching the same levels as for men. There has been a general upgrading of the workforce over time; there was a decrease in the numbers of both male and female unskilled workers although women still constituted a larger share (54%) than men (46%) of unskilled workers in 2000.

The gender difference in level of participation in paid work narrowed as women abandoned the housewife role (35% of women in 1968) and entered the labour market, although often as part-time workers (49% in 1981, 36% in 2000). Fewer men were full-time workers in 2000 (70%) than in 1968 (84%). Household responsibility also became more evenly shared between men and women. The female share of this responsibility was 91% in 1968 and 57% in 2000.

There were significant changes in gender differences for all work environment factors included between the years 1981 and 2000, when people outside the labour market were excluded (Table 3.2). Women's ergonomic load significantly increased whereas there was no change among men. A considerably smaller

Figure 3.1(a)-(d): Gender-specific development of musculoskeletal pain and psychological distress and gender differences (women–men) in three age groups (1968-2000)

(a) Prevalence of musculoskeletal pain

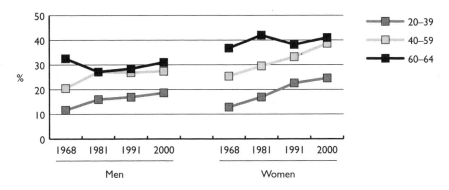

(b) Prevalence of psychological distress

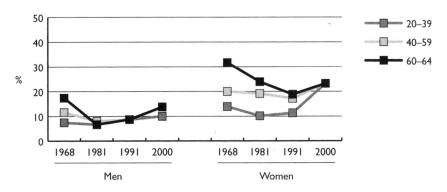

(c) Gender differences in musculoskeletal pain **(d) Gender differences in psychological distress**

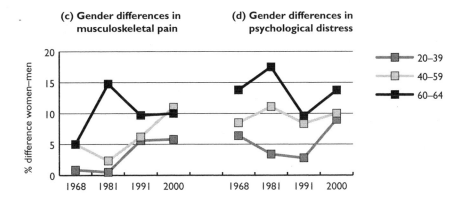

Table 3.2: Age standardised distribution of work environment factors for gainfully employed men and women aged 20-64[a] and proportion of women in each category in 1981 and 2000 respectively (%)

	Men		Women		% women in group	
	1981	2000	1981	2000	1981	2000
Ergonomic load				*		
Low	28	25	27	21	45	44
Medium	46	48	51	54	49	50
High	26	28	21	26	40	46*
Physical/chemical load		*		*		
Low	28	37	45	49	58	54
Medium	35	29	47	42	54	56
High	37	33	8	9	15	19*
Psychological demands		*		*		
Low	29	23	29	18	45	41
Medium	37	37	42	36	49	46
High	34	39	29	46	42	51*
Varied work						
No	16	19	20	19	51	47
Yes	84	81	80	81	45	48*
n	1,978	1,811	1,673	1,629		

Note: [a] Age standardised by the direct method and five-year age groups. The age distribution in the entire sample for all periods was used as the reference population.

* Change between 1981 and 2000 significant ($p < 0.05$) as indicated by χ^2-test.

proportion of women than men were exposed to a high physical/chemical load, although there was a significant improvement for men over time. Moreover, high psychological demands rose from 29% to 46% for women while for men the increase over the period was only from 34% to 39%. Similarly high proportions of men and women judged their work to be varied.

There are marked age differences in how full-time paid work has changed for men and women. The proportion of women in full-time work has increased throughout the period for 40- to 59-year-olds and 60- to 64-year-olds but decreased for 20- to 39-year-olds between 1991 and 2000 (Figure 3.2). For men, there was a fall in the proportion of full-time workers in all age groups after 1968. Changes in part-time work have been relatively similar across age groups among women and for men aged 60-64 (an increase followed by a decrease), while it rose somewhat for men aged 20-39 and 40-59. The increase in 'no paid' work between 1991 and 2000 was greatest among men aged 60-64 and women aged 20-39 (which rose by 14 and 12 percentage units respectively) and smallest among women aged 60-64.

Figure 3.2: Development of full-time, part-time and 'no paid' work for men and women in three age groups (1968-2000)

(a) Full-time work

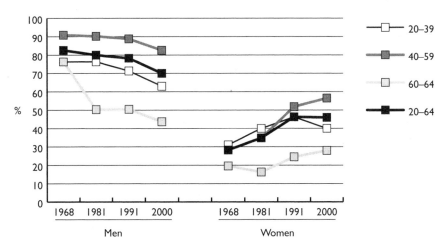

(b) Part-time work

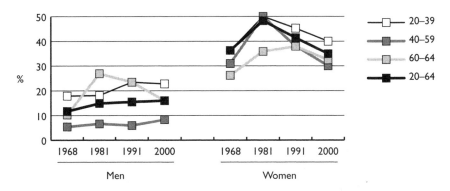

(c) 'No paid' work

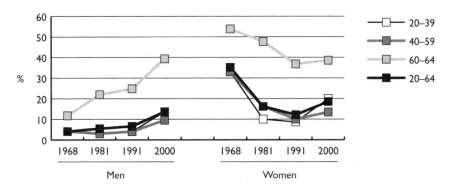

Determinants of gender differences in musculoskeletal pain

Two important criteria must be fulfilled when we analyse the changing contribution of various factors to gender differences in ill health: (1) the association between an independent (risk) factor and the health outcome; and (2) the gender difference in this factor. Over time there have been changes in both of these. As regards the first, a number of risk factors were found to be significantly related to musculoskeletal pain in only one or two of the four periods (adjusted for age and gender): living alone (1991); children at home (1981 and 1991); social network (1991 and 2000); and household responsibility (2000).

There was an historically fairly stable pattern (Table 3.3) for the factors that clearly contribute to women's excess in musculoskeletal pain over men's (own income and psychological distress), those that tend to contribute a small amount or nothing (marital status, living alone, children at home, socioeconomic status) or in a reversed direction (social network). Paid work was an important contributor in 1968 but *not* in later periods (Table 3.3, model 8 compared to model 1). Household responsibility contributed to women's excess musculoskeletal pain in 1968 and in 1981 (in particular), but less so in 1991 and 2000 (model 9). In all periods, own income was the most important factor for gender differences in musculoskeletal pain, and its inclusion in the logistic regression models (model 6) made the odds ratios (OR) insignificant in 1968 and 1981, and changed from 1.39 to 1.17 in 1991 and from 1.56 to 1.31 in 2000. Similar effects were observed when psychological distress was added to the regressions (model 10).

If we turn to the contribution of work environment factors, analysed for 1981 and 2000 only (Table 3.3, models 11–14), monotonous work was of importance for women's excess pain in 1981 whereas high chemical/physical load contributed in an opposite direction in 1981 and 2000. An equalisation of such risks would lead to larger gender differences in musculoskeletal pain than those that were actually observed. When factors most clearly found to contribute to gender differences in musculoskeletal pain are included simultaneously, namely own income and psychological distress (model 15) and when household responsibility, that was important in the beginning of the period, was added (model 16), the OR tended to indicate no significant gender differences in 1968 and 1991, a slight male excess in 1981 (OR 0.78 [0.62–0.98]) and a slight female excess in 2000 (1.16 [1.00–1.36]). Considering exposure to chemical and physical risks, which are more prevalent among men, there were no gender differences in musculoskeletal pain in 1981, and a clearly significant female excess in 2000 (model 17).

Determinants of gender differences in psychological distress

Nearly all social factors included were found to be of significance for psychological distress in all observation years (not shown in a table). Household responsibility (not significantly associated with psychological distress in 1981) and age (unrelated

Table 3.3: Period-specific gender differences (women relative to men) in musculoskeletal pain adjusted for various factors (1968, 1981, 1991 and 2000)

Models	1968 OR (95% CI)	1981 OR (95% CI)	1991 OR (95% CI)	2000 OR (95% CI)
1 Age	1.23 (1.06-1.43)	1.16 (1.01-1.35)	1.39 (1.20-1.60)	1.56 (1.36-1.79)
2 Age + marital status	1.21 (1.04-1.42)	1.14 (0.98-1.32)	1.38 (1.19-1.59)	1.53 (1.34-1.76)
3 Age + lives alone	1.23 (1.06-1.43)	1.17 (1.01-1.35)	1.40 (1.21-1.61)	1.56 (1.36-1.79)
4 Age + children at home	1.23 (1.06-1.44)	1.17 (1.01-1.35)	1.39 (1.21-1.60)	1.55 (1.35-1.78)
5 Age + social network	1.24 (1.06-1.44)	1.19 (1.03-1.38)	1.40 (1.22-1.62)	1.59 (1.38-1.82)
6 Age + own income	0.93 (0.77-1.12)	0.94 (0.79-1.10)	1.17 (1.00-1.36)	1.31 (1.13-1.51)
7 Age + socioeconomic status	1.21 (1.03-1.43)	1.14 (0.98-1.33)	1.37 (1.18-1.59)	1.54 (1.34-1.78)
8 Age + paid work	1.08 (0.90-1.31)	1.12 (0.95-1.33)	1.40 (1.21-1.63)	1.49 (1.29-1.72)
9 Age + household responsibility	1.17 (0.90-1.51)	1.04 (0.84-1.28)	1.37 (1.18-1.59)	1.51 (1.31-1.73)
10 Age + psychological distress	1.04 (0.89-1.22)	1.02 (0.88-1.18)	1.26 (1.09-1.46)	1.36 (1.18-1.57)
11 Age + ergonomic load	–	1.14 (0.98-1.33)	–	1.55 (1.35-1.78)
12 Age + chemical/physical job load	–	1.37 (1.17-1.61)	–	1.76 (1.52-2.03)
13 Age + psychological. job demands	–	1.10 (0.95-1.28)	–	1.50 (1.31-1.72)
14 Age + varied work	–	1.08 (0.93-1.25)	–	1.54 (1.34-1.77)
15 Age + own income + psychological distress	0.87 (0.72-1.05)	0.86 (0.72-1.01)	1.10 (0.94-1.29)	1.19 (1.02-1.38)
16 15 + household responsibility	0.85 (0.64-1.12)	0.78 (0.62-0.98)	1.11 (0.94-1.31)	1.16 (1.00-1.36)
17 16 + chemical/physical job load	–	0.97 (0.76-1.22)	–	1.38 (1.17-1.62)
n	4,525	4,287	4,220	4,274

to the outcome in 2000) were exceptions. Household responsibility was related to less psychological distress in 1968 (adjusted for age and gender) and to more such distress in 1991 and 2000. The opposite association in 1968 should be interpreted with great caution because there was multi-collinearity between gender and household responsibility in 1968 (0.78), and controlling for gender makes any general conclusion for this variable in 1968 problematic.

Although the social determinants of psychological distress differ from those of musculoskeletal pain, own income seemed also to be the most important contributing factor to gender differences in psychological distress. Including income led to lower OR for all periods (Table 3.4, model 6 compared to model 1). Paid work in all periods (model 8), socioeconomic status in 1981 (model 7) and musculoskeletal pain in 2000 (model 10) also made a considerable contribution (a fall in the OR by at least 0.15). For a number of factors, women were in more favourable social circumstances than men, thus leading to increased OR; this was because women were more likely than men to have children at home (model 4) and a high level of social networks (model 5). Women were also more likely to be married (1981 and 2000, model 2) and consequently less likely to be living alone (1981 and onwards, model 3).

Work environment factors in the form of high ergonomic load, high psychological demands and monotonous work contributed to women's excess in psychological distress in 1981, but less so in 2000 (Table 3.4, models 11-14). It is important to observe that this contribution mainly stems from the 'no work' category in the work environment variables, and that we could not assign work environment exposure to those without a work environment.

A relatively large share of women's excess psychological distress can be attributed to own low income and less involvement in the labour market in all observations, but clearly most in 1968 (Table 3.4, model 15). When musculoskeletal pain (men favoured) and social network (women favoured) are also included, the female excess was about 50% in 1968 and 1991, double in 1981 and 70% in 2000 (model 16). In a final model, which added household responsibility, the gender differential in psychological distress became clearly smaller in 1991 (as compared to model 15), somewhat smaller in 1981 and 2000, but clearly greater in 1968 (model 17).

Gender-specific associations between work and health outcomes

In the period 1968-2000 associations between degree of labour force participation and the two health outcomes changed from being gender-specific to having more gender-equal associations (Figure 3.3). Men who were excluded from the labour market in 1968 had extremely high levels of psychological distress compared to full-time workers. The health gap (OR) between non-working men and those in full-time positions fell from about 9 to 2.5. An opposite development occurred for psychological distress among women, that is, there was a widening health gap between non-working women and those working

Table 3.4: Period-specific gender differences (women relative to men) in psychological distress adjusted for various factors (1968, 1981, 1991 and 2000)

Models		1968 OR (95% CI)	1981 OR (95% CI)	1991 OR (95% CI)	2000 OR (95% CI)
1	Age	2.13 (1.79-2.55)	2.33 (1.90-2.85)	1.79 (1.47-2.18)	1.97 (1.68-2.31)
2	Age + marital status	2.08 (1.74-2.50)	2.38 (1.94-2.93)	1.79 (1.47-2.19)	2.01 (1.71-2.37)
3	Age + lives alone	2.13 (1.78-2.54)	2.39 (1.94-2.93)	1.85 (1.52-2.25)	2.04 (1.74-2.39)
4	Age + children at home	2.16 (1.80-2.58)	2.37 (1.93-2.91)	1.83 (1.50-2.23)	1.99 (1.69-2.33)
5	Age + social network	2.25 (1.88-2.70)	2.45 (1.99-3.02)	1.92 (1.57-2.34)	2.08 (1.77-2.45)
6	Age + own income	1.41 (1.14-1.75)	1.75 (1.39-2.19)	1.42 (1.15-1.76)	1.65 (1.40-1.95)
7	Age + socio-economic status	2.11 (1.75-2.55)	2.15 (1.74-2.66)	1.67 (1.36-2.04)	1.93 (1.64-2.28)
8	Age + paid work	1.50 (1.21-1.87)	1.95 (1.55-2.45)	1.64 (1.33-2.02)	1.82 (1.54-2.14)
9	Age + household responsibility	2.51 (1.87-3.35)	2.20 (1.64-2.96)	1.62 (1.32-1.99)	1.90 (1.62-2.24)
10	Age + musculoskeletal pain	2.10 (1.75-2.53)	2.30 (1.87-2.84)	1.65 (1.35-2.02)	1.80 (1.53-2.12)
11	Age + ergonomic load	–	2.14 (1.74-2.65)		1.93 (1.64-2.27)
12	Age + chemical/physical job load	–	2.33 (1.86-2.92)	–	1.99 (1.68-2.35)
13	Age + psychological. job demands	–	2.12 (1.72-2.62)	–	1.87 (1.59-2.20)
14	Age + varied work	–	2.00 (1.62-2.46)	–	1.94 (1.65-2.28)
15	Age + own income + paid work	1.32 (1.05-1.65)	1.80 (1.42-2.28)	1.47 (1.19-1.83)	1.68 (1.42-1.99)
16	15 + social network + musculoskeletal pain	1.50 (1.19-1.90)	1.96 (1.54-2.50)	1.51 (1.20-1.90)	1.68 (1.40-2.01)
17	16 + household responsibility	1.91 (1.39-2.62)	1.90 (1.38-2.61)	1.34 (1.06-1.70)	1.65 (1.37-1.98)
n		4,525	4,287	4,220	4,274

Figure 3.3: Age-adjusted gender-specific associations between degree of labour force participation and musculoskeletal pain and psychological distress, 1968 to 2000: men and women aged 20-64

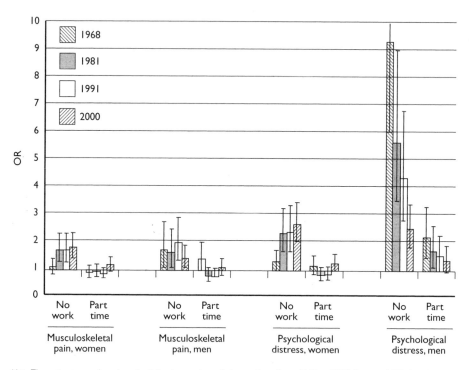

Note: The estimates are based on the following number of observations (from 1968 to 2000) for men 2,303, 2,180, 2,150, 2,210; and for women 2,248, 2,133, 2,079, 2,082.

full time, in particular in the period 1968-81. For women this development was similar for musculoskeletal pain and psychological distress. For both health outcomes in all survey years, the health of women working part time has been no poorer than that of women working full time. From 1991 and onwards, men and women had similar risks of psychological distress and musculoskeletal pain in the same labour force participation group.

We did find changes in gender differences in particular for musculoskeletal pain in the period 1968-2000. We therefore focus here on the significant increase in women's excess musculoskeletal pain. The modelling presented in Table 3.3 does not tell us which factors have caused the increase in this gender differential. It is a paradox that as gender differences in own income have considerably narrowed towards the smallest differences in 2000, the gender gap in musculoskeletal pain was the greatest. Moreover, men still tend to be more exposed to heavy physical job demands and risks. Here, however, a narrowing is likely to be related to the increased prevalence of pain among women and a stable or declining prevalence among men. We therefore wanted to analyse possible gender-specific effects of

Figure 3.4: Age-adjusted gender-specific associations between ergonomic load and musculoskeletal pain in 1981 and 2000 (OR compared to those with low ergonomic load)

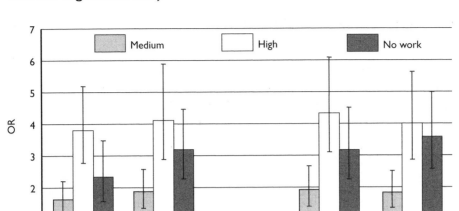

ergonomic load, since these seemed to be the most important factors for musculoskeletal pain.

There were strong associations between ergonomic load and musculoskeletal pain for both men and women (Figure 3.4). A high ergonomic load was somewhat more strongly related to pain than was having no paid work, which suggests that a shift from having a high ergonomic load to 'no work' could be related to an improvement in musculoskeletal pain. Simultaneously, such shifts are likely to increase the level of such pain for the group with 'no work'.

It is of methodological importance that there tended to be gender-specific associations between own income and musculoskeletal pain as well as psychological distress in certain survey years but not in others. Own income was more strongly related to female than male musculoskeletal pain in 2000: men in income quintiles 1 through 4 had OR between 1.30 (quintile 1, insignificant estimate) and 2.08 (quintile 2) compared to men in the highest income quintile, whereas the corresponding estimates for women were in the range 1.59 (quintile 4) and 3.42 (quintile 2). Income was also insignificant in relation to women's psychological distress in 1968 and 1991 (not shown in a table).

Conclusion

We found that gender differences had significantly widened (in an absolute as well as a relative sense) for musculoskeletal pain but persisted for psychological distress over a 32-year period of generally narrowing gender differences in factors such as labour force participation, own income, work environment factors and household responsibility.

Explanations for changing health differentials

It may appear paradoxical that Swedish welfare policies aiming for gender equality over the period under study have not resulted in smaller health differences between men and women. Changes believed to be beneficial for women's health, in particular increased labour force participation and number of hours worked by women (and a corresponding decrease in labour force participation and number of hours worked by men), have led to stable gender differences in psychological distress and growing gender differences in musculoskeletal pain. This simplification of the long-term development became more complex after 1991. The Swedish recession in the 1990s resulted in an increase in economic inactivity due to unemployment. However, women aged 40-59 and 60-64 were more likely to be in full-time employment in 2000 than in 1991, something that was not the case among men and women aged 20-39. One interpretation of this development is that the process of women entering the labour market on equal terms with men should be seen as a slow process that has not yet finished. About one third of Swedish women still work part time in 2000, and *only* 38% of full-time workers in Sweden were women in 2000 compared to 25% in 1968. It should be mentioned that most part-time working women in Sweden, including those with children, work at least 26 hours per week rather than 15 hours or less, which is common in many other European countries (Montanari, 2001). Nevertheless, the slow improvement in the share of women in the highest income group is therefore a logical consequence not only of the fact that women have low-paid jobs, but also that they work a lower number of paid hours than men.

A large number of previous studies which aim to 'explain' gender differentials in morbidity indicators have found that the explanatory variables included in their analyses only partly explain such differentials (for example, Nazroo et al, 1998; McDonough and Walters, 2001; Walters et al, 2002; Denton et al, 2004). This is particularly true for psychological distress. Some studies have shown that gender differences vary greatly across age groups and health outcomes (Macintyre et al, 1996). Gender differences in own income and participation as well as in number of hours of paid work clearly contribute to gender differences in psychological distress in all observation periods. A number of social factors are more favourable to women, such as having a well-developed social network and children in the home. However, women's greater involvement in social networks does not seem to be substantially protective of their psychological wellbeing compared to men.

Two factors were clearly found to contribute to gender differences in musculoskeletal pain in all survey years: own income and psychological distress. The change towards greater equality in own income is the opposite of the change in gender differences in musculoskeletal pain. A large study based on a Swedish county found that the numbers of pain conditions reported were strongly related to psychiatric problems, but to the same extent for men and women (Bingefors and Isacson, 2004). One Finnish sample of middle-aged women suggests that there is also a strong association between physical health and depressive symptoms (Aro et al, 2001). Similar findings have been reported from Britain and Sweden (Popay et al, 1993; Ringbäck Weitoft and Rosén, 2005). The order of causality here is not clear, but it has been shown that simultaneously suffering from a number of common symptoms, physical and mental, is an expression of stress, especially among women (Krantz and Östergren, 1999). Although there was greater co-morbidity between psychological distress and musculoskeletal pain among women than among men, this did not change over time, and has probably not contributed to the greater increase in female relative to male pain.

The changes in working conditions for men and women, and the number of hours exposed to these conditions, have probably been important for changes in musculoskeletal pain. After 1981, the male work environment tended to improve more than the female one. This is in line with other Swedish studies (Lidwall et al, 2004). Ergonomic load is among one of the most important factors for developing musculoskeletal pain (Volinn and Punnett, 2001; Aittomäki et al, 2005). Over time it became more common for women than for men to work in jobs with a medium or high ergonomic load. Moreover, at the same time women aged 40-64 increased their time spent in paid work. They were therefore probably more exposed to health hazards from paid work in 2000 than in 1991. This development could have contributed to some of the increased gender differences in musculoskeletal pain, at least among the middle-aged. A more detailed analysis of particular male and female working conditions might help us to establish why there has been a clear increase in women's reporting of musculoskeletal pain relative to men's in the past 25 years. We might look at possible interaction effects between physical and psychosocial working conditions for the development of musculoskeletal pain (Volinn and Punnett, 2001).

Gender-specific experiences

The puzzling finding of greater gender equality but increased or stable health differences between men and women raises the question of whether there could be gender-specific associations between social and economic factors and the health outcomes studied here. Furthermore, it is likely that health effects of a social factor (such as being unemployed) changes over time, and perhaps not in the same way for men and women. Bingefors and Isacson (2004) found that being married and having economic difficulties were related to prevalence of pain for women but not for men. We also observed that a number of factors did not relate to men and women in the same way, such as paid work and own income. In 1968, the health of women outside the labour market was not poorer than that of those who were gainfully employed. By 2000, non-working women and men tended to have significantly poorer health than labour force participants and the gender differences in musculoskeletal pain and psychological distress did not seem to vary greatly between the categories of full time, part time or economically inactive. It is more difficult to evaluate the finding of changes in how own income is associated with male and female psychological distress and musculoskeletal pain. The contribution of income to women's higher prevalence of musculoskeletal pain in 2000 assumes that there are roughly similar associations between income and pain for men and women. The fact that income was not as strongly associated with male as compared with female musculoskeletal pain in 2000 suggests that an analytical approach that only focuses on trying to find gender differences in exposure variables has limitations, and that a number of factors are not related to men's and women's illness symptoms in the same way. This could be due to the largely different characteristics of typically female and male work, not least the monetary rewards from the job. It could also be due to the fact that the association between ergonomic load (a factor that showed similar associations with men's and women's pain) and own income differs between men and women.

It is possible that the 'double exposure' experienced by women who work full time, that is, holding a demanding job and shouldering a high work burden in the home (Hall, 1992; Artazcoz et al, 2001; Krantz et al, 2005), has resulted in the increased workload of paid work counteracting the possible benefits of any improvements achieved in paid work. We did find significant gender differences in musculoskeletal pain, with women reporting more pain than men among full-time workers, in 1968, 1991 and 2000, but not in 1981 (not shown in a table). The observation of no gender difference in musculoskeletal pain among full-time workers in 1981 does not give full support to the hypothesis of double exposure. Neither does the finding that gender differences in musculoskeletal pain were as large among those outside the labour force as among those working full time in 2000. This does not correspond with the hypothesis that women are more susceptible to musculoskeletal pain when exposed to adverse working conditions. It has been suggested that an adverse psychosocial work environment could be related to musculoskeletal pain over and above physical work factors (van den Heuvel et al, 2005), something that we could not analyse in a satisfactory way here due to the inclusion of economically inactive men and women. Job strain is clearly more prevalent in female than in male work settings (see Chapter Five).

A gender-specific association between age and pain has been found among the gainfully employed in a Finnish study (Aittomäki et al, 2005). We found the same interaction: there was a significant association between age and pain among women but not men in the age group 40-59 and 60-64. As in the Finnish study, we observed that ergonomic load declined with increasing age among men but not among women. The likelihood of retiring early on a disability pension is higher for women than for men after at least 1986 (Hemström, 2001a), and musculoskeletal disorders account for a greater share of female than male early retirement on a pension in 2000 (Hemström, 2002). Therefore, an absent gender-specific effect of ergonomic load on pain could be underestimated due to the healthy worker effect, in the sense that there has been a greater selection of women than of men with pain into a non-work situation. Similar explanations were suggested in a study that found no effect of duration of employment in the current job on musculoskeletal pain for women, but a significant such effect for men (Dahlberg et al, 2004).

Limitations of the study

The study has a number of limitations that need to be discussed. One is the possibility that there is a systematic gender bias in how respondents answer questions on health symptoms, and whether the two health measures are comparable for the whole period from 1968 to 2000. If there are indeed significant gender differences in response to questions about health, it is less clear whether there have been changes in gender differences in reporting poor health in surveys, and whether there are significant differences in such gender-specific reporting for psychological distress and musculoskeletal pain. Although a number of studies have found that women tend to over-report their ill health in surveys, in particular minor morbidity (Verbrugge, 1989), others suggest either the opposite or only small such differences (Macintyre, 1993; Macintyre et al, 1999). In a meta-analysis of experimentally induced pain, the possibility that men tend to be socialised to under-report pain is discussed (Riley et al, 1998). It also reported that a number of studies have identified physiological factors that possibly make women more sensitive to pain than men. The phenomenon of women's higher prevalence of musculoskeletal pain is most likely multidimensional.

The present study focuses more on factors related to paid work than to unpaid household duties. This is because the most major change in living conditions to occur during the period in question was women's entry into the labour market. Unfortunately, items on household activities were not measured adequately for the entire period, and such items were not included at all in 1968. The measure we did use, household responsibility, is far from optimal. It is difficult to evaluate whether the narrowing gender gap in running a household has been similar as regards the time spent on various unpaid home duties.

Conclusion of the study

This study aimed to examine whether any changes took place over a 32-year period in gender differentials in musculoskeletal pain and psychological distress – the two most common reasons for certified sickness absence in Sweden among both women and men. We found an increased gender differential in musculoskeletal pain after 1981 and a fairly stable gender differential in psychological distress in the entire period 1968-2000, although living conditions (socioeconomic and psychosocial factors) became more equal for women and men over the period. Moreover, it became obvious that the changes observed for gender differences in musculoskeletal pain could only partially be attributed to changes in those social factors included in this study, of which own income and psychological distress contributed most.

Of the factors studied here, own income and paid work contributed most to gender differences in psychological distress. We found some variation in the factors that contributed to gender differences in the two health outcomes analysed here, and we also found a great variation in how various factors were related to psychological distress on the one hand and musculoskeletal pain on the other. When men's greater exposure to physical and chemical work factors were taken into consideration, women had significantly more musculoskeletal pain than men in 2000. The unfavourable development of musculoskeletal pain in women after 1981 (and for 40- to 59-year-old women in particular) is, we believe, due to one or more of the following: (1) increasing adverse conditions in female workplaces along with improvements in male workplaces; (2) an increasing proportion of women aged 40-64 working full time; (3) women continuing to have the main responsibility for unpaid household tasks and childcare, that is, a high total work burden which gives rise to stress and ill health in at least certain periods of life.

FOUR

Life course inequalities: generations and social class

Johan Fritzell

Introduction

This chapter studies health inequalities from a generational perspective but also aims to adopt a life course perspective. The interest in generations lies with the fact that birth cohorts encounter specific historical conditions and circumstances, situations that deviate from those of both earlier and later generations. 'Children of the great depression' is but one famous example in the literature (Elder, 1974). The life course approach further emphasises the dimension of time from the individual's perspective by, for example, focusing on the long-term consequences of specific historical conditions encountered earlier in life.

No one can deny that the historical and social circumstances that we encounter when new born or in youth have an immediate impact on our lives. At the same time it seems likely that both short- and long-term consequences have a socioeconomic dimension. For example, although the immediate problem of trying to get into the labour market during a recession is obvious, it seems plausible that there are also substantial class deviations both with regard to difficulties in finding a job and perhaps also how well you are able to cope without one. In epidemiological terms it could be said that both the exposures to circumstances, such as unemployment, and vulnerability, or susceptibility, in terms of how exposure in turn increases the risk of ill health, are likely to vary depending on your class background. The focus of attention in this chapter is class inequalities in health as formed by the close relation to age and generation.

Discussions about generational inequalities seldom address the interrelation between class and generation. In life course approaches to human development there is, of course, a long tradition of distinguishing attitudes and behaviour within working-class and middle-class families (see, for example, Moen et al, 1995), but there is less focus on how class differentials in certain outcomes vary between generations. This chapter specifically tries to grasp how class divisions in health have changed across generations. While class differentials can be studied from several angles, a fundamental distinction is between class of origin and class of destination. From a perspective of generational belonging it seems natural to focus in particular on class of origin. In other words, to what extent the social position of your parents is of importance for your health in later life, and to what degree this association has changed for individuals born in different generations. A question to be asked first is therefore: when we look at class differentials in health from a generational perspective do we then find any equalisation? When examining this topic from the perspective of childhood class, this question can be rephrased as dealing with changes in *equality of opportunity* (for health).

In life course epidemiology it is common to discuss and possibly measure accumulation of risk (Ben-Shlomo and Kuh, 2002). In simple terms, such a model supposes that the impact on health of inferior conditions, or exposure to health risks, accumulates over the life course. A simple, but complicated enough, model of this kind is to try to differentiate class of origin and adult class position to study the independent, simultaneous and cumulative effect on a health outcome, sometimes also including class of first job (see for example, Davey Smith et al, 1997). This approach does indeed enhance our understanding of which phases seem to be of greatest importance for the risk of ill health and perhaps in particular highlights different patterns for different diseases. Competing theories, however, are not always possible to disentangle (Hallqvist et al, 2003). I will take advantage of a specific feature of our data, namely a work-life history section, which makes it possible to model the *time* spent in various class positions (for a thorough description and analyses of the biography sections in the Level-of-Living Surveys [LNU], see Jonsson and Mills, 2001). By simultaneously studying how social origin, present adult class position and the cumulative class experience influence health outcomes the following question is posed: does cumulative class experience contribute to health inequalities over and above present (and childhood) class position?

The chapter begins with a discussion of some important topics related to generations and the life course approach. In essence, much of this debate focuses on the pertinent question of time. This is followed by a section on data, and the construction of key variables. The empirical section starts by presenting some background data on class differences in mortality by birth cohort. The analyses that follow focus not only both on childhood class inequalities for different birth cohorts across various parts of the life course, but also how these differentials relate to adult class position. The final part of the empirical section presents results that focus on how ill health is differentiated depending on a person's total class experience in life so far. This is followed by a discussion of how to interpret the findings.

Generating generational differences across the life course

In order to be interested in differences between generations, there is one basic prerequisite, namely, social change. In a static society, those of a specific age will be in the same situation as an older generation when they were at the same age. Conversely, it has often been suggested that the study of generations is an excellent way of understanding social change (Ryder, 1965; Alwin, 1992). Although this is more commonly discussed in political sociology and attitudinal research, the idea of 'cohort replacement theory' surely has the potential to be relevant in many other fields.

It seems likely that the experience of dramatic events, such as war or famines, will have consequences for the long-term health of those alive at the time and this is supported by research findings (for example, Sparén et al, 2004). The effect on population health is, however, not always what one would expect. As noted by Sen (1995), life expectancy in Britain had its fastest increases during the two world wars. Sen notes that this apparent paradox was most probably brought about by effective redistributional policies and how scarce resources were allocated. Indeed, Richard Titmuss, as early as 1950 (see also Alcock et al, 2001), discussed at length how the rationing of food, coupled with a number of specific social reforms and full employment, had a powerful impact on vital statistics during the Second World War.

Yet less dramatic events and social circumstances can also be of relevance. An influential theory about birth cohorts has to do with mere size. Generational size, following periods of baby booms and low birth rates, is expected to be of great influence on your life chances and living conditions. According to the 'Easterlin hypothesis', larger cohorts will generally be disadvantaged precisely due to numbers. Members of a large birth cohort will face stronger competition when they enter the labour market; this will, in turn, reduce their relative wages and, according to the theory, strongly affect their social and demographic behaviour. They will marry at a later age and have a lower fertility rate (Easterlin, 1980). Although highly influential, the empirical support for this theory has varied somewhat (Pampel and Peters, 1995).

The generations to be studied here have indeed experienced different social circumstances. On the macro-structural level one could argue that we should expect diminishing class differentials due to the development and maturation of the Swedish welfare state. Many of the social reforms of the 20th century have undoubtedly had the double overarching aims both of generally improving life and of equalising life chances and living conditions.

A specific and classic problem in all generational or cohort analyses is that there is an exact mathematical identity between cohort, period and age. Period is the sum of birth year and age. Therefore it is impossible to estimate all these factors unless you have some restrictions in your model strategy. Nevertheless, a generational analysis can often shed new light on findings that are usually seen in too simple an age perspective.

Critical periods and accumulation

The life course approach in epidemiology distinguishes the critical period from accumulation of risk. In short, critical period refers to a window of time in an individual's life when an exposure will have an especially strong, or even irreversible, health impact in the long run. As discussed by Ben-Shlomo and Kuh (2002), the critical period model exists both in a stronger and softer version. The extent of irreversibility and the issue of time are of great importance for this distinction. The stronger version implies that an adverse event will necessarily lead to a certain outcome, whereas the softer version can be seen as implying that events happening later on in life may change or modify the effect of the earlier exposure.

This softer version bears more similarities to the idea of an accumulation model in which one sees the total duration of health hazards as the most important feature – a certain period may anyway be seen as more influential than others. Childhood is often seen as an important period of this kind. In Sweden, as elsewhere, childhood conditions have been seen as exerting an influence on adult morbidity and mortality (Vågerö and Leon, 1994; Lundberg, 1997). It should be noted that the influence of childhood versus that of other periods of life is likely to vary depending on which specific outcome we are considering. This is also the general conclusion of a recent review of the relation between socioeconomic circumstances during childhood and adult mortality (Galobardes et al, 2004).

Those studying life course epidemiology have shown a great interest in the accumulation hypothesis. This hypothesis predicts, in terms of social position, that the negative health influence of a disadvantaged position ought to be stronger the longer the duration is. While such a statement appears plausible, few studies have actually studied the effect of total class experience. Kåreholt (2001) used the same data as that used in this chapter to explore a time-varying social class but did not focus on the accumulation in the same manner as here. A recent article by Ljung and Hallqvist (2006) has a similar strategy to the one adopted here, and suggests that not only duration but also temporal ordering might be of importance.

Of course the relative scarcity of studies with this approach is partly due to lack of data. In social sciences in general a classic example is the labour market and mobility study of Oakland more than 50 years ago. In that study, wage earners reported detailed histories of job shifts and occupation. From that data source Lipset and Bendix (1952, 1959) calculated the proportional time spent in various class positions. Tåhlin (1987) made a similar approach with Swedish data.

Although neither of these studies analysed health, their findings underline that it is hard to predict what to expect in terms of health inequalities between social classes. The total class experience is likely to be of some importance but might very well be captured by present class. Tåhlin (1987), for example, found that unskilled workers, the category with the most stable position, had close to 90% of their accumulated job experience in their present class. If one focuses on what is sometimes labelled the holding power of classes it is, instead, strongest in the upper strata. In other words, if you manage to climb to a higher position the chances of staying there are very great. At any rate, the relatively high degree of stability could very well imply that a measurement of total class experience will have no explanatory power over and above that of present position in the social structure. This is by and large what Tåhlin concluded when studying a number of political attitudes. On the other hand, in a study with British data, Power et al (1999), using one of the health outcomes to be studied in this chapter (self-rated health [SRH]), concluded quite the reverse: "... *duration* of exposure to socioeconomic conditions has a strong predictive effect on health status" (p 1062, original emphasis). A further question is to what extent we should expect life course pattern and outcome to vary from one nation or welfare regime to another (for example, Mayer, 2001).

While the accumulation hypothesis may be correct from a theoretical standpoint, it presupposes a certain amount of intra (or inter)-generational social mobility, on the one hand, in order to be of any empirical importance. If this is the case it poses, on the other hand, the difficult question of health-related social mobility versus social causation (Illsley, 1955; Lundberg, 1991; Elstad, 2004). Moreover, it also introduces the possibility that social mobility per se is related to health.

Crucial measurement questions

The perspective taken in this chapter involved using a number of LNU surveys; in other words, information was collected from a number of years. This means that time interferes with our crucial measurements. Because of this it is necessary to give a brief account of how this was dealt with in the empirical analysis.

Class measurement

The measurement of social class is central to the analysis. In this case several important choices and distinctions were involved, because the analysis deals both with time, the usual crux of how to operationalise class, and which class differentials to emphasise. To start with the time dimension, the first empirical sections present class differentials with the help of childhood class and adult class, while the last empirical section will study time, or rather share of life, spent in different classes, including childhood and employment history in adult life. This will be explained in more detail when the empirical results are presented.

In accordance with other chapters in this book, occupation and the Swedish socioeconomic classification are used as the basis for measuring class. Class of origin will be based on main occupation of the father. An admittedly crude categorisation will be used throughout this chapter. Class of origin or adult class position will be defined according to the simplest but also most crucial dividing lines in the class structure. Thus, we will separate non-manual from manual workers, but will also in most instances report farmers and self-employed people separately. There are several reasons for this broad classification. Firstly, it simplifies the presentation while keeping the basic division between manual and non-manual occupations. Secondly, the statistical power would become too weak if we used a refined class categorisation within each birth cohort. Thirdly, the changes in job content in a more finely-graded occupational structure would be likely to lead to greater problems with comparability when comparing someone born at the beginning of the 20th century with the current situation.

Our data enables us, however, to also include a more direct measure of childhood condition. In addition to class of origin, an indicator of economic hardship during childhood will also be used. This indicator is based on one question that reads: 'Did your family suffer from economic difficulties during your upbringing?' with a simple 'Yes' or 'No' as response alternatives. Despite the simplicity of this indicator, it has proved to be of importance for adult health status (Lundberg, 1993).

Although the same concept and categorisation of class and the same indicator on economic hardship are used throughout the analysis, we still encounter inherent comparability problems. One of them is related to class structure. Like most other countries, Sweden saw profound changes in class structure in the 20th century, as we mentioned in Chapter Two. Two great waves of change are particularly notable. Firstly, Sweden industrialised quite late and thus the farming class remained a large category for most of the 20th century. Today it is a negligible segment of the working population, yet not so in terms of class of origin. The second great wave was the structural changes involved in the transition from industrial to post-industrial society, with an increasingly larger fraction of the labour force becoming non-manual employees, especially in employment related to services. The other side of this coin is the decline in the proportion of manual workers, as we reported in Chapter Two.

These are not merely compositional changes in the class structure; they are also related to changes in the character of work. Bell (1973) put it well when he wrote that pre-industrial work is a game against nature, industrial work is a game against fabricated nature and machines, while in post-industrial societies work is primarily a game between people. These compositional and characteristic changes might also influence our findings, a topic we will come back to in the concluding discussion.

Classification of generations

A second important question refers to the categorisation of generations. Ideally one should aim for a theoretically driven principle so that specific historical circumstances would guide the analysis, as exemplified by 'children of the great depression'. However, it is not self-evident exactly which societal changes and experiences in the past should be regarded as the most influential; neither do we have a precise understanding of when during the life span the impact of a historical event is greatest (for an excellent discussion on 'timing' in this respect, see Elder, 1995). Moreover, we do not have the ideal data for such a categorisation. Instead I choose a parsimonious solution, with generations being defined according to the decade in which a person was born, that is, people born in the 1930s, 1940s and so on. This is also the solution used in earlier studies based on data from the

LNU surveys (for example, Hörnqvist, 1994). However, a further complication is that we only have health status for survey years and that the time interval between surveys varies a little. The irregularity of the surveys means that total comparability across birth cohorts is not possible. Although the data include health measurement covering more than 30 years, we obviously cannot compare class differentials in health at the same age for people born in, say, 1910 with those in 1970s. It is, nevertheless, possible to analyse the extent of class inequality in different generations across part of the life course, and it is this possibility that will be explored.

Health indicators

In the first part of our analysis we will study class differential by musculoskeletal pain as well as the broader summed index presented in Chapter Two. *Musculoskeletal pain* is measured by questions about aches in shoulders, pain in back or hips, and pain in hands, elbows, legs or knees. *High symptom load* is constructed from 42 specific items following the question: 'Have you in the last 12 months had any of the following illnesses or ailments?'. For each of the 42 items the respondent answers 'No', 'Yes, mild' or 'Yes, severe'. The index is dichotomised so that those answering at least 'Yes, severe' to two of these illness (or 'Yes, mild' on at least six items) are classified as being ill. Questions about *SRH* were only asked in the two most recent LNU surveys (conducted in 1991 and 2000). Therefore this measure is not used in the first broad part of the analysis. However, some partial analysis comparing adjacent birth cohorts will be performed. SRH will also be used as an outcome in the second part of the empirical section dealing with the effect of total class experience, together with analyses of musculoskeletal pain.

Analytical strategy

I have purposely chosen a very parsimonious strategy in the analyses to come. Accordingly, the analyses will not include more proximal intervening mechanisms, such as health behaviours, in order to understand the causal process in more detail. There are a number of reasons for this choice. Firstly, the aims and research questions in this chapter have a different character. Secondly, in line with the proponents of the idea that social class is a basic or fundamental cause (Lieberson, 1985; Phelan et al, 2004), it is not self-evident that we always get a greater causal understanding by including a number of other independent variables. Thirdly, in my opinion, the idea of linking more proximal factors to a more distal cause, like social class, makes more sense when studying specific diseases. As we discussed at length in Chapter One, the health indicators used in this book tend to be of a more general character. Of course this is not to say that rigorous attempts to study complex chains should be avoided.

Empirical results

The main focus of attention in this chapter is on various forms of ill health. As a counterpart it seems natural to say something about class differentials in mortality for various birth cohorts. Accordingly Figure 4.1, calculated from a demographic study by Statistics Sweden (2002) based on population statistics, reports class differentials in expected average years of life between the ages 20 and 85 by birth cohort for women and men separately. The staples reflect differentials between non-manual and manual workers expressed in average years. For example, men belonging to the non-manual classes, born in 1950 or 1955, had an average life expectancy from age 20 of about 60.5 years. The corresponding figure for manual workers was just under 58 years. The difference between the two (2.8 years) is reported in the figure. Simple as these figures are, they are based on a rather complicated model aiming to predict future mortality based on current trends comparing adjacent five-year birth cohorts.

In line with what was described in Chapter Two, these staples show that class has far from lost its importance in people's life chances. For women we find that class differentials are clearly on the rise. It is less clear for men but the average yearly difference is nevertheless higher for those born in the 1950s than for those born in the 1930s. For the country internationally known as something of a world champion in equality these figures are indeed interesting, or perhaps even embarrassing. Of course, what is not seen in the figure is that life expectancy has increased for men and women of both classes, but the increase is indeed

Figure 4.1: Differences in life expectancy (average years) between 20 and 85 years of age for non-manual and manual workers among women and men born in the 1930s, 1940s and 1950s, respectively

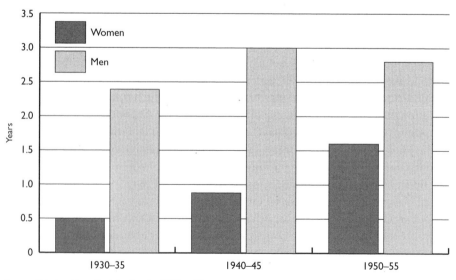

Source: Calculated from Statistics Sweden (2002, p 13)

small among working-class women. As was mentioned in Chapter One, this widening of the gap between lower and higher social positions seems to be a common experience for many western societies (Crimmins and Saito, 2001; Marmot, 2004; Mackenbach, 2005a).

Influence of class of origin

To what extent, then, are various forms of ill health related to childhood class, and is it fully mediated by present adult class? Figure 4.2 depicts *absolute* differences in prevalence of musculoskeletal pain by class of origin for six different birth cohorts at different ages. Childhood class is dichotomised so that we compare individuals from non-manual origin to others. Since Chapter Three scrutinised gender differentials in part from a birth cohort perspective, I have chosen to report results from an analysis in which women and men are collapsed. All analyses are also performed stratified by gender, and notable gender differences will be commented on. Despite the fact that our outcomes are measured over several decades, it is impossible to carry out a full comparison over the whole life course across birth cohorts, as the presented curves clearly reveal.

If we look at prevalence differences for pain (Figure 4.2), we can note a number of general features, despite the rather scattered picture presented. First, we note that they are generally fairly modest in younger ages, increase sharply in middle-age and then tend to decrease as people reach retirement age. This pattern of how class differentials in health vary over the life course appears to be a typical finding (House et al, 1990). What is specific here is that class is defined by class

Figure 4.2: Absolute differences in the prevalence of musculoskeletal pain between individuals born of manual workers or farmers/self-employed versus non-manual class for six different birth cohorts by age

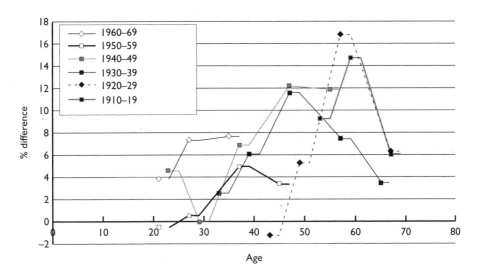

of origin. Nevertheless, it is fascinating that family background becomes more and more important over the life course (up to retirement age), but it partly reflects the intergenerational transmission of inequality and the strong determinants of social position by childhood position.

What, then, does Figure 4.2 tell us about differences between birth cohorts? It is not totally unambiguous but in one of birth cohorts (1950s), the differences are particularly small. It is tempting to see this as a general feature of higher equality of opportunity, which in turn could be related both to more general modernisation processes and to welfare state development and expansion. This interpretation is, however, complicated by the fact that the curve for those born in the 1960s is clearly above that seen for the preceding cohort. This difference between individuals born in the 1960s compared to those born in the 1950s is apparent when these cohorts are around 20 years of age and remains when they have reached the age of about 35. I will return to this birth cohort difference later in the chapter.

We then come to more specific analyses in which we compare birth cohorts at specific ages, including present adult class position. Are the differences shown in Figure 4.2 wholly accounted for by the strong influence of class of origin on one's own class position as an adult? Do we find a similar pattern across birth cohorts for adult class position as the one we found for childhood class? These are questions we now turn to by making more specific comparisons of birth cohorts at certain ages and also including the other measure of childhood conditions, namely economic hardship.

Table 4.1 presents results from a number of logistic regressions for three birth cohorts, namely those born in the 1930s, 1940s and 1950s. For all birth cohorts our data refers to the situation at around 45 years of age. Consequently, the data used comes from different waves of the LNU. Table 4.2 reports results from similar analyses but now for birth cohorts at around 65 years of age. The cohorts in this table were born in the 1910s, 1920s and 1930s. The dependent variables are musculoskeletal pain and high symptom load. The tables present crude and mutually adjusted estimates for class of origin, self-assessed economic hardship during upbringing and present class position. All models are further controlled for gender. Non-manual workers are, as before, used as reference category, but the class variables now distinguish three categories, namely non-manual workers, manual workers and farmers/self-employed people. Non-significant estimates are not reported but since the statistical power is quite low in these regressions the tables present estimates if they are 'significant' on a 10% level.

If we look at the situation among the middle-aged (Table 4.1), and starting with the generation born in the 1930s, we find a more than double excess risk for manual workers with regard to pain and a slightly lower excess risk for high symptom load for the 1930s generation. Childhood class is also clearly associated with the risk for both outcomes but this effect is partly mediated by own class position. It is also notable that people with their upbringing in the group of farmers and/or self-employed in fact have the highest excess risk both for the

Table 4.1: Odds ratios (OR) for musculoskeletal pain and high symptom load, crude and mutually adjusted by class of origin and present adult class position for three different birth cohorts at ~45 years of age[a]

	Musculoskeletal pain		High symptom load	
	Crude	**Mutually adjusted**	**Crude**	**Mutually adjusted**
	OR (95% CI)	OR (95% CI)	OR (95% CI)	OR (95% CI)
Birth cohort 1950-59				
Childhood class				
Non-manual	1.00	1.00	1.00	1.00
Manual workers	ns	ns	ns	ns
Self-employed, farmers	ns	ns	ns	ns
Childhood economic hardship				
No	1.00	1.00	1.00	1.00
Yes	ns	ns	2.09 (1.40-3.10)	2.03 (1.35-3.05)
Adult class				
Non-manual	1.00	1.00	1.00	1.00
Manual workers	1.35 (1.00-1.82)	1.34 (0.99-1.83)	1.47 (1.09-1.97)	1.41 (1.04-1.92)
Self-employed, farmers	ns	ns	ns	ns
	n = 928		n = 928	
Birth cohort 1940-49				
Childhood class				
Non-manual	1.00	1.00	1.00	1.00
Manual workers	1.87 (1.28-2.72)	1.55 (1.05-2.28)	1.34 (0.95-1.90)	ns
Self-employed, farmers	2.13 (1.43-3.17)	1.79 (1.19-2.69)	1.44 (0.99-2.08)	ns
Childhood economic hardship				
No	1.00	1.00	1.00	1.00
Yes	ns	ns	1.56 (1.11-2.21)	1.53 (1.07-2.19)
Adult class				
Non-manual	1.00	1.00	1.00	1.00
Manual workers	2.03 (1.53-2.70)	1.88 (1.40-2.52)	1.70 (1.29-2.24)	1.61 (1.21-2.14)
Self-employed, farmers	1.45 (0.92-2.29)	1.45 (0.92-2.29)	ns	ns
	n =1,071		n = 1,071	
Birth cohort 1930-39				
Childhood class				
Non-manual	1.00	1.00	1.00	1.00
Manual workers	1.94 (1.19-3.16)	ns	1.51 (0.98-2.31)	ns
Self-employed, farmers	2.25 (1.38-3.67)	1.75 (1.05-2.92)	1.87 (1.22-2.87)	1.58 (1.01-2.46)
Childhood economic hardship				
No	1.00	1.00	1.00	1.00
Yes	2.55 (1.84-3.55)	2.47 (1.75-3.47)	2.01 (1.46-2.76)	2.00 (1.44-2.78)
Adult class				
Non-manual	1.00	1.00	1.00	1.00
Manual workers	2.27 (1.63-3.17)	2.02 (1.43-2.87)	1.70 (1.26-2.31)	1.61 (1.17-2.22)
Self-employed, farmers	1.66 (1.01-2.73)	1.49 (0.89-2.49)	ns	ns
	n = 834		n = 834	

Note: [a]All models controlled for sex

ns =non significant

Table 4.2: Odds ratios (OR) for musculoskeletal pain and high symptom load, crude and mutually adjusted by class of origin and present adult class position for three different birth cohorts at ~65 years of age[a]

	Musculoskeletal pain		High symptom load	
	Crude	Mutually adjusted	Crude	Mutually adjusted
	OR (95% CI)	OR (95% CI)	OR (95% CI)	OR (95% CI)
Birth cohort 1930-39				
Childhood class				
Non-manual	1.00	1.00	1.00	1.00
Manual workers	1.72 (1.08-2.73)	ns	ns	ns
Self-employed, farmers	1.54 (0.95-2.47)	ns	1.80 (1.16-1.78)	1.59 (1.01-2.50)
Childhood economic hardship				
No	1.00	1.00	1.00	1.00
Yes	2.07 (1.44-2.98)	1.91 (1.30-2.81)	2.12 (1.47-3.07)	2.11 (1.43-3.11)
Adult class				
Non-manual	1.00	1.00	1.00	1.00
Manual workers	2.27 (1.61-3.19)	2.04 (1.43-2.90)	1.70 (1.23-2.36)	1.52 (1.08-2.14)
Self-employed, farmers	ns	ns	ns	ns
	n = 648		n = 648	
Birth cohort 1920-29				
Childhood class				
Non-manual	1.00	1.00	1.00	1.00
Manual workers	ns	ns	ns	ns
Self-employed, farmers	ns	ns	ns	ns
Childhood economic hardship				
No	1.00	1.00	1.00	1.00
Yes	ns	ns	1.51 (1.08-2.10)	1.38 (0.97-1.95)
Adult class				
Non-manual	1.00	1.00	1.00	1.00
Manual workers	1.85 (1.28-2.67)	1.81	1.42 (1.02-1.99)	ns
Self-employed, farmers	ns	ns	ns	ns
	n = 668		n = 668	
Birth cohort 1910-19				
Childhood class				
Non-manual	1.00	1.00	1.00	1.00
Manual workers	ns	ns	1.47 (0.94-2.31)	ns
Self-employed, farmers	ns	ns	1.77 (1.13-2.76)	1.57 (0.97-2.53)
Childhood economic hardship				
No	1.00	1.00	1.00	1.00
Yes	2.06 (1.50-2.83)	1.96 (1.41-2.73)	1.89 (1.39-2.56)	1.88 (2.53-2.58)
Adult class				
Non-manual	1.00	1.00	1.00	1.00
Manual workers	1.70 (1.16-2.48)	1.44 (0.95-2.18)	1.39 (1.00-1.96)	ns
Self-employed, farmers	ns	ns	1.47 (0.96-2.24)	ns
	n = 768		n = 768	

Note: [a]All models controlled for sex

ns = non significant

1930s and 1940s cohorts. The more direct indicator of economic hardship during childhood is also quite strong and seems to be relatively uninfluenced by the class measures. While by and large the findings are quite similar for people born in the 1930s and 1940s, they are not reproduced for the youngest cohort in the table. Here we find that childhood class is already non-significant in the crude model. The direct indicator of childhood condition is also non-significant, but only with regard to pain. The estimates also indicate a much weaker effect of present class position for people born in the 1950s. While it is evident that the effects of childhood class mainly work through the adult class position in these analyses, the same is not true for our more direct measure of economic hardship during upbringing.

In Table 4.2 the estimates with regard to pain are more often insignificant or, if significant, lower than in Table 4.1. This reflects to some extent what we saw in Figure 4.2; this pattern also appears to be valid for adult class position. This finding seems to indicate, in accordance with one theme in life course research generally, that class differentials in health vary over the life course, and that these differences widen particularly in mid-life but then gradually decline somewhat (House et al, 1990). Or, it might more simply be a question of generally higher prevalence in older age, which often tends to reduce differences in terms of odds ratios (OR). It is important to stress that from the data presented here it is not possible to identify to what extent this reflects a general age pattern profile since it could also reflect cohort-specific patterns.

Otherwise, many of the general patterns are reproduced for the older birth cohorts. For the birth cohorts of the 1910s and 1920s the effects of our childhood measures are surprisingly small. Selection bias might be a problem here, since a non-negligible proportion of people born in these generations have died before reaching this age (65), and this risk is higher in the lower classes. However, it might also reflect more real processes. Diderichsen and Dahlgren (1991) have previously reported surprisingly small social differences in mortality for these birth cohorts, especially among people born in the 1910s, which does not lend any support to the social selection explanation.

The results presented so far indicate that the influence of class of origin to a large extent works through adult class position. From the birth cohort perspective one might suggest that the generation of the 1950s marks a new break, in that it seems hard to find any significant influences of class of origin. Although from these data one cannot rule out the possibility that it is just is a question of time, it seems likely to reflect a true difference compared with the two preceding generations.

As we have noted previously, SRH cannot be used as an outcome covering a longer time perspective since this more global measure has only been included in the two most recent LNU surveys. In other words, for each birth cohort we have only two snapshots in time of SRH over the life course. Nevertheless, we can make some comparison between adjacent pairs of birth cohorts. Table 4.3 reports the results of regressions similar to those carried out earlier but now with

SRH as the dependent variable and concentrating on the younger cohorts, since we are particularly interested in the results for the generation born in the 1950s. We thus compare this generation with that born in the 1960s at around the age of 35, and with that born in the 1940s at around the age of 45.

Once again we find that childhood class is not significantly related to the outcome for those born in the 1950s, whereas the crude association is quite strong for those born in the 1940s. It is also evident that this influence works largely through own class, while the opposite is true for childhood economic hardship, in line with previous analyses in this chapter. Those born in the 1960s have a very similar outcome to the preceding cohort both with respect to childhood class and own class. However, economic hardship during upbringing is also significant in the mutually adjusted model. When one looks at these

Table 4.3: Odds ratios (OR) for SRH less than good, crude and mutually adjusted by class of origin and present adult class position: pairwise birth cohort comparisons at age ~35 and ~45[a]

	Crude	Mutually adjusted	Crude	Mutually adjusted
	OR (95% CI)	OR (95% CI)	OR (95% CI)	OR (95% CI)
At age ~35	**Birth cohort 1960-69**		**Birth cohort 1950-59**	
Childhood class				
Non-manual	1.00	1.00	1.00	1.00
Manual workers	ns	ns	ns	ns
Self-employed, farmers	ns	ns	ns	ns
Childhood economic hardship				
No	1.00	1.00	1.00	1.00
Yes	1.93 (1.26-2.95)	1.80 (1.15-2.81)	ns	ns
Adult class				
Non-manual	1.00	1.00	1.00	1.00
Manual workers	1.83 (1.30-2.56)	1.69 (1.18-2.42)	1.91 (1.29-2.84)	1.94 (1.28-2.94)
Self-employed, farmers	ns	ns	ns	ns
	n = 1,023		n = 949	
At age ~45	**Birth cohort 1950-59**		**Birth cohort 1940-49**	
Childhood class				
Non-manual	1.00	1.00	1.00	1.00
Manual workers	ns	ns	1.56 (1.02-2.37)	ns
Self-employed, farmers	ns	ns	1.73 (1.11-2.69)	ns
Childhood economic hardship				
No	1.00	1.00	1.00	1.00
Yes	1.85 (1.22-2.79)	1.74 (1.14-2.67)	2.16 (1.50-3.12)	2.09 (1.42-3.07)
Adult class				
Non-manual	1.00	1.00	1.00	1.00
Manual workers	1.76 (1.27-2.44)	1.72 (1.23-2.42)	2.40 (1.74-3.31)	2.27 (1.62-3.18)
Self-employed, farmers	ns	ns	ns	ns
	n = 924		n = 1,070	

Note: [a]All models controlled for sex

ns = non significant

relations among earlier generations (at older ages) a very similar pattern appears to that reported for the 1940s cohort in Table 4.3 (the results for the older generations are not shown in the table). In other words, there is a clear indication of the influence of class of origin; in the mutually adjusted models this effect becomes non-significant, whereas the overall size of the excess risk for manual workers is quite large and declines only marginally when childhood conditions are adjusted for.

Thus, when we adjust for adult class position, childhood class becomes non-significant in almost all cases. On the contrary, and as expected, manual workers have significantly higher odds for musculoskeletal pain, for having a high symptom load and for rating their health as poor. In most cases this higher prevalence is not markedly reduced by adjusting for childhood class. In a recent study of Swedish males born around 1950, Hemmingsson and Lundberg (2005) found that childhood and conditions in youth 'explained' most of the increased risk for coronary heart disease (CHD) hospitalisation and mortality among employed workers. This result is definitely not repeated here, but on the other hand Hemmingsson and Lundberg included not only childhood class but also a number of lifestyle factors at younger ages. Nevertheless, it is rather remarkable that we see such small changes in the estimates for own class when we adjust for childhood class. At the same time it should be noted that in almost all analyses presented so far we find that the indicator of economic hardship during upbringing is significantly related to various forms of ill health. One should obviously not interpret the findings for the crude measure of childhood class as implying that family background is irrelevant.

One focus of attention in these analyses has been the issue of changing class differentials across generations. What conclusions can we draw thus far? Most of our analyses indicate relatively modest class inequalities for the oldest birth cohorts (1910s and 1920s), after which there is a shift in the pattern and it seems that for people born in the 1930s and 1940s class differentials are especially strong. A new shift seems to occur for those born from the 1950s and onwards – not in the sense that class differentials as such have disappeared when studied on the base of adult present occupation, although they seem to be slightly lower than earlier. A more qualitative change is that class of origin has lost in importance. Class of origin is often regarded as the key marker for chances in life. In that sense *equality of opportunity* to have a decent health status seems to have progressed in Sweden.

Accumulation of class experience

Let us now move to the question that can be said to be at the heart of the life course approach in relation to social stratification. Such an approach, as previously pointed out, starts from the idea that social outcomes that we observe at a specific point in time are not just explained by contemporaneous factors but are the result of the accumulation of living conditions and processes occurring during the whole life span. In relation to class differentials, both generally and with regard to health outcomes specifically, this implies that one's position in the social structure both today and in the past is of importance. Even though this idea seems plausible, relatively few attempts have been made to model the full class career. The common empirical approach has instead been to investigate this question by simultaneously including some indicator of class (or some other socioeconomic indicator) during upbringing and present class position in a similar way to what was done earlier in this chapter. The lack of studies that model the full career is definitely not a result of lack of interest but rather of the fact that few datasets allow for a more finely-graded test of this topic.

As was mentioned previously, the results of any such attempts are a bit ambiguous because people's class position is relatively stable. This might lead us to conclude that present class position, possibly together with class of origin, is empirically able to sum up any accumulated effects. It is important to stress that such a result does not necessarily mean that there is anything wrong with the hypothesis as such. Such a result could well be due to the inertia of the social structure.

Here, I calculate total class experience using a very simple but central division in the class structure, namely the basic distinction between non-manual and manual employment, or, more precisely, singling out non-manual positions versus all other positions. Our key variable is one that originates in retrospective work-history biographies starting with the first regular job of at least six months' duration. Class of origin is also incorporated into the measurement. Here, the data, in line with earlier, permits just one classification that aims to identify the main class position during the first 16 years of life. Accordingly, the degree of class changes is somewhat under-estimated in the analysis.

Since our respondents are of different ages the final variable is calculated as the *share* of total life that each individual has spent in non-manual classes. The measure thereby varies between 0 and 1. For example, a woman has a working-class background; she starts working at the age of 16 and has a number of jobs as a shop assistant. However, from the age of 30 until the age of 41 she works as a clerk. Her company then closes and at the time of the interview she is 44 years old and has been in and out of employment (only unskilled manual jobs) for the past three years. This person has in total 11 years within the non-manual category, which equals 0.25 (11/44) in our measurement of accumulated time as a non-manual worker.

Not surprisingly, we get a measure with a very peculiar distribution; about a third of the sample have a value of 0, whereas around 10% were born into the non-manual category and have stayed there all their lives so far. The latter have a value of 1 on our accumulated time variable. The main empirical question is to what extent can such a measure capture more variation in the dependent variable compared to the more standard version in the life course approach, that is, class of origin and present class position?

Due to data constraints our measurement of health status refers now only to the 1991 survey and includes people born in the 1940s and 1950s. At the time of measurement the people in these cohorts were consequently between 32 and 51 years of age. A few individuals without any job experience lasting for six months were excluded from the analysis. The accumulated time variable is, somewhat arbitrarily, divided in five categories with the '0 category' being the largest one. The reference category consists of those with more than 90% of their class experience within non-manual classes. Because of possible multi-collinearity between the different class variables I refrain from presenting a full model that includes childhood class, adult class and the variable measuring accumulated class experience. Instead the comparison will be made between one model that includes the two former variables, and another that solely includes the accumulated class experience.

Table 4.4 presents results of a number of logistic regressions with SRH and musculoskeletal pain as the outcomes. Starting with the results for SRH, we see that the crude models of childhood class and present class, respectively, show results quite as expected. Both are clearly significant, the OR of having poor SRH increases by close to 50% for those not coming from non-manual classes, whereas the parameter estimate for present class position is nearly double in strength. When we mutually adjust for childhood class and present adult class both coefficients decrease a little but reach significance. The estimates for the accumulated class experience suggest a stronger relation. The OR is slightly above 3 for those with no time in non-manual classes, whereas it sinks to slightly

Table 4.4: Odds ratios (OR) for SRH less than good and musculoskeletal pain by childhood class, present adult class and accumulated class experience: men and women aged 32-51, class divisions between non-manual workers and others[a]

	SRH less than good		Musculoskeletal pain	
	Crude	**Mutually adjusted**	**Crude**	**Mutually adjusted**
	OR (95% CI)	OR (95% CI)	OR (95% CI)	OR (95% CI)
Childhood class				
Non-manual	1.00	1.00	1.00	1.00
Others	1.48 (1.09-2.00)	1.29 (0.95-1.77)	1.66 (1.28-2.15)	1.47 (1.13-1.92)
Present adult class				
Non-manual	1.00	1.00	1.00	1.00
Others	1.93 (1.50-2.49)	1.86 (1.43-2.41)	1.90 (1.53-2.36)	1.80 (1.44-2.23)
Accumulated time experience in non-manual classes				
0		3.15 (1.90-5.23)		3.93 (2.52-6.12
0.01-0.30		2.12 (1.20-3.77)		2.37 (1.44-3.91)
0.31-0.60		1.31 (0.75-2.27)		1.90 (1.19-3.03)
0.61-0.90		1.47 (0.82-2.63)		1.84 (1.12-3.03)
0.91-1		1.00		1.00
n		1,896		1,897

Note: [a] All models adjusted for age and sex.

above 2 for those with at most 30% of their experience in such positions, all in relation to the reference category.

When we turn to the analysis of the risk of musculoskeletal pain the results are even stronger. The OR for childhood class and present adult class are approximately in the same order as for SRH, although slightly higher for childhood class. The estimates for the accumulated variable is, however, clearly stronger here. In both cases, other model statistics also suggest that the accumulated class experience has a better fit with the data.

To further test this conclusion the effect of an interaction variable between childhood and adult class was modelled. The OR was about 2 and 2.3 (not seen in the table) comparing those in the 'others' position in both cases versus those who were in the non-manual classes both during childhood and at present. This can, roughly, be contrasted with the 3.15 and 3.93 estimates presented in Table 4.4, consequently confirming the conclusion that the measurement of the accumulated class experience managed to capture more of the health variation both with regard to musculoskeletal pain and SRH.

Women and men are collapsed in the analysis presented in Table 4.4. Gender stratified analyses, however, indicate much stronger effects for men than for women (not seen in the table). This was also partly the case in earlier analyses although less marked. A plausible reason for this discrepancy between men and women is that we have used own occupation as the basis for classification rather than a family-based measure of social position (see Erikson, 2006). This gender difference does not, however, change the general conclusion since the measure of accumulated class experience performs better for both women and men.

Of course, one should be careful and somewhat cautious about interpreting these results; we deal with only two health outcomes, have a very crude, although important, class division, with a sample of individuals quite early and in the middle of working life in Sweden. However, in no respect do these facts, in my mind, lead to a bias that would favour the measurement of total class experience. At any rate, the results indeed indicate that we are able to make a more stringent distinction with the accumulated class variable compared to our standard measures.

Conclusion

This chapter has scrutinised class differences in a number of health outcomes from the perspectives of generational belonging and the life course. The main findings were the following. Firstly, even though the main preoccupation in this chapter has been ill health as opposed to mortality, an indication of widening class differentials in life expectancy was presented. This was shown when looking at successive birth cohorts. This is a finding in line with what we presented for age groups in Chapter Two. Secondly, in more recent birth cohorts, class of origin seems to have lost in importance for several health outcomes. This is indicative of an increase in equality of opportunity which, in my mind, is of great importance. In so far as we found effects of class of origin it works to a very large extent through present class position. Thirdly, clear evidence of a strong impact of childhood condition was found with regard to the direct measure of economic hardship during upbringing. These effects worked largely over and above class (as measured here). Family background, more generally, clearly has a strong health impact in adulthood. Fourthly, present adult class, according to almost all the analyses, strongly influences the risk of ill health. Fifthly, the accumulation hypothesis received clear support in that a variable measuring total class experience across life has a closer and stronger relation to ill health than do present and childhood class.

Of course these findings should be regarded with caution. Due to the relatively small number of observations in some of the cohort-specific analyses the statistical power is fairly weak. In particular some non-significant estimates, for example with respect to effects of class of origin, may be due to this. Because of the statistical power problem I used very crude measures of social class, basically just dividing non-manual and manual workers. While this was necessary when analysing separate birth cohorts, a more refined measurement of class would surely have captured more health differentials. The changing class and job structure, as well as the strong educational expansion, are likely to influence the results when one compares across birth cohorts.

More theoretically, to distinguish effects of childhood class and present class is difficult. As so eloquently proved by Elstad (2001), the relations between these, and the effects they produce in a statistical model, are strongly influenced by compositional changes and in particular by social mobility and social selection. However, in so far as we find no effect at all of childhood class this problem does not exist. Consequently I tried in particular to base my conclusions on such findings.

With regard to the accumulation hypothesis, future research should also look at the temporality and direction of class changes, not just the total experience as such. It seems likely that upward social mobility might have different effects than downward mobility. Moreover, one should in detail analyse when during the life course these effects are especially strong in line with the critical period discussion previously mentioned.

Despite these caveats and the obvious shortcomings of the analyses I hope to have indicated that the life course approach is a fruitful way of analysing how health differentials between classes are produced, changed and reproduced. The chapter also provides a theoretical linkage between macro-social conditions and micro-level analysis.

FIVE

Work stress and health: is the association moderated by sense of coherence?

Susanna Toivanen

Introduction

This chapter focuses on whether personality characteristics, in terms of sense of coherence (Antonovsky et al, 1990; Sagy et al, 1990), may buffer against the adverse effects of work stress exposures. To see why this research question is interesting, it is essential to recall the dramatic economic development in Sweden during the 1990s. The recession was severe with obvious consequences for the labour market, working conditions and people's lives.

Unemployment hit high levels; in 1993 8.2% of the labour force was out of work (Figure 5.1). The rising unemployment level had an impact on working conditions. Consequently, many of those still employed faced a higher risk of ill

Figure 5.1: Employed as % of the Swedish population, 16-64 years; unemployed as % of the labour force, 16-64 years (1990-2000)

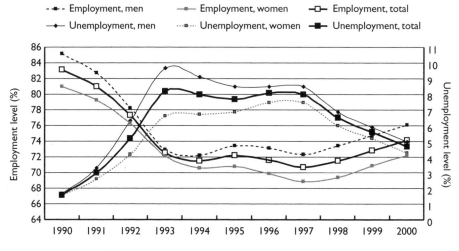

Source: Statistics Sweden (2005c)

health and psychosocial problems due to aggravating circumstances at work. Physical working conditions, described as physically demanding and monotonous work, remained relatively stable during the decade. However, the risk of having a physically demanding job was higher for women (Fritzell et al, 2000b). Work intensity changed; the share of job strain (a combination of high psychological demands and low decision latitude) increased. This increase in job strain was unequally distributed in the population, with the highest increase within the public sector (le Grand et al, 2001). During the second part of the decade, the expenses for sickness absence started to rise in an uncontrollable manner that resulted in considerable costs for the welfare state (SOU, 2002, p 5). The increase was highest for long-term sickness absence, and the share of stress-related ill health escalated (Näringsdepartementet, 2000). Even if Sweden has a strong tradition of reforms and research in the field of working conditions, these important questions were not on the agenda during the times of economic depression in the early 1990s. The escalating sickness absence levels in the late 1990s brought the issue of work stress once more into focus (Tåhlin, 2001).

Two broad lines of research can be distinguished in the field of occupational stress: (1) the stress related to exposure to physical hazards at work, and (2) the stress related to exposure to psychosocial hazards. Physical hazards may be of biological, biomechanical, chemical and radiological character (Cox et al, 2000). Various physical hazards interact with one another, and with psychosocial hazards, to create effects on health (Schrijvers et al, 1998). For example, adverse physical working conditions in combination with psychosocial work stress were found to increase the risk of musculoskeletal disorders (Vingård et al, 2000). Psychosocial aspects of work in relation to employees' health have been studied since the early 1950s. At the beginning the focus was mostly on individual differences in adaptation and coping, and how these individual aspects influenced employees' health. Since the 1960s the focus has shifted towards the design and management of work as a cause of work-related ill health (Cox et al, 2003). An influential model in this field is the demand-control model that postulates that high psychological demands in combination with low decision latitude at work may have detrimental effects on health (Karasek, 1979; Karasek and Theorell, 1990).

However, quite recently the focus of occupational stress research in Sweden seems to be turning towards factors related to work and private life that are associated with long-term good health among employees (Aronsson and Lindh, 2004). Inspired by this line of research the present chapter aims at investigating whether sense of coherence may moderate the effect of physical and psychosocial work exposures on health. The salutogenic model suggested by Antonovsky (1987a) focuses on factors that promote good health. Sense of coherence partly explains why individuals are able to resist stress and maintain good health while experiencing adverse circumstances. Thus, sense of coherence is a crucial factor when dealing with stress. It is assumed that a strong of sense of coherence may determine successful coping with adverse working conditions (Antonovsky, 1979). Previous research has showed that a strong sense of coherence seems to protect workers from strain and thus maintain wellbeing in work-life settings (Kalimo et al, 2002, 2003).

Nevertheless, the moderating role of sense of coherence on the effects of work stress on health has not been investigated prospectively using a representative sample of the Swedish working population. The Level-of-Living Surveys (LNU) for 1991 and 2000 give a unique opportunity to test this hypothesis in a population sample by combining the salutogenic model with work stress exposures assessed by physical demands and the demand-control model. However, before investigating the moderating role of sense of coherence, it is crucial to explore whether there is a predictive association between the two work stress exposures or sense of coherence or both, and the health outcomes. In this chapter the analyses focus on psychological distress and musculoskeletal pain since these are the main conditions associated with long-term sickness absence during the 1990s (Lidwall and Skogman Thoursie, 2000). Hence, these two conditions impair the quality of life for the employed individuals, and burden welfare resources. Because the Swedish labour market is segregated by gender (Nermo, 1999), gender differences will also be under scrutiny.

Research questions

This chapter focuses on the following research questions:

- First, was there any change in work stress exposures, in sense of coherence, or in the prevalence of psychological distress and musculoskeletal pain between 1991 and 2000? Are there gender differences in these factors?
- Second, does work stress exposure or a weak sense of coherence or both predict psychological distress or musculoskeletal pain incidence?
- Third, does a strong sense of coherence moderate the work stress effect on psychological distress or musculoskeletal pain?

Background

Physical demands

Exposure to physical demands may affect health through a direct physical pathway or a psychological stress-mediated pathway or both (Cox et al, 2000). Worrying that physical demands might be detrimental to health may evoke fear and anxiety that may lead to impairments in psychological health in the long run (Levi, 1984; Cox et al, 2000). Thus, exposure to physical demands may affect both psychological and physical health. The physical demands of work often found as risk factors for musculoskeletal disorders include heavy lifting, forceful exertion, twisting, and non-neutral body postures (Holmstrom et al, 1992; Ekberg et al, 1994; Hoogendoorn et al, 2000; Häkkänen et al, 2001; Feveile et al, 2002; Punnett et al, 2004). Some people question the work-relatedness of musculoskeletal disorders and claim that the causes of such health impairments could also be non-occupational. However, the available epidemiological evidence on the work-relatedness of musculoskeletal disorders is substantial (Bernard, 1997). The etiologic importance of occupational ergonomic exposure, such as physical demands, for the occurrence of musculoskeletal disorders of the lower back and upper extremities has been demonstrated (Punnett and Wegman, 2004).

Demand-control model

A well-known theoretical instrument for assessing psychosocial work stress is the demand-control model created by Karasek (1979). The model was later developed in cooperation with Theorell (Karasek and Theorell, 1990), and also expanded to include social support (Johnson, 1986). According to the demand-control model, the combination of psychological demands and decision latitude at work determines the effect of psychosocial work stress on employees' health and wellbeing. These combinations give four specific work situations: active (high demands and high decision latitude), job strain (high demands and low decision latitude), passive (low demands and low decision latitude), and low strain (low demands and high decision latitude). The two main hypotheses of the demand-control model are the strain hypothesis and the buffer hypothesis. According to the former, job strain may lead to psychological and physical illness in the long run. However, the buffer hypothesis postulates that high decision latitude may moderate the adverse effects of high demands on health. In addition, it is hypothesised that social support moderates the adverse effects of job strain (Johnson, 1986; Karasek and Theorell, 1990).

Decision latitude (job control) comprises two components: decision authority and skill discretion. Decision authority is a socially agreed form of control over job performance. This means that the employee can decide how and when the job is done. Skill discretion refers to control over the use of one's skills in the job. It is implied that decision latitude is unequally distributed in modern organisations since the highest level of knowledge legitimises the exercise of the highest level of authority. According to Karasek and Theorell, decision authority and skill discretion are closely related theoretically and empirically and are therefore usually combined (Karasek and Theorell, 1990, 2000). Psychological demands refer to 'how hard you work', and include factors related to time pressure, mental stimulation and coordination responsibilities. Physical demands are not reflected by the demand-control model, even though physical exertion is likely to be a source of mental arousal. Working hard includes high physical demands for many groups of workers. The assessment of psychological demands is methodologically problematic since questions about psychological demands are understood differently by different groups, for example, men and women, and manual and non-manual workers (Karasek and Theorell, 2000; see also Kristensen et al, 2004).

The demand-control model has been studied in association with a large number of health outcomes and mortality (see, for example, Schnall et al, 1994; Belkic et al, 2004; Job Stress Network, 2005). The model has been employed in relation to psychological outcomes such as burnout (Bourbonnais et al, 1998), psychological distress (Bourbonnais et al, 1998; Vermeulen and Mustard, 2000), and work-related psychological wellbeing (de Jonge et al, 2000a). The results are relatively consistent, indicating that job strain is associated with impairment of psychological health. However, the moderating effects of decision latitude and social support on the adverse effects of job strain have not yielded consistent results, possibly due to the limited number of studies, and inconsistency in the conceptualisation of the demand–control model across empirical studies (van der Doef and Maes, 1999).

Regarding the association between the demand–control model and musculoskeletal pain, low job control was found to be related to shoulder disorders in supermarket cashiers (Niedhammer et al, 1998), and job strain increased the risk of musculoskeletal disorders in transit operators (Rugulies and Krause, 2005). According to a review of psychosocial work stress in relation to musculoskeletal disorders, there is evidence that high demands at work are associated with upper extremity problems such as musculoskeletal pain. To a lesser extent, this association was also valid for poor control at work (Bongers et al, 2002). A review of psychosocial factors and neck pain found some evidence for a positive relationship between both high demands and low job control and neck pain (Ariëns et al, 2001).

Sense of coherence

The salutogenic model of sense of coherence emerged from Antonovsky's (1979, 1987a) studies on holocaust survivors. Antonovsky wondered how some people remained healthy despite devastating conditions. He proposed that every individual has internal and external resistance resources that facilitate dealing with different kinds of stressors in everyday life. The internal resistance resources include factors such as intelligence, knowledge and social competence. The external resistance resources include social support from other people, sound working conditions, adequate material resources, and cultural and social factors. Having sufficient internal and external resistance resources, and being able to use these resources in an advantageous way, was found to be a key to successful coping with stressful conditions. Thus, sense of coherence is defined as a global orientation towards one's inner and outer world (Antonovsky, 1979, 1987a).

Sense of coherence is based on three components labelled comprehensibility, manageability and meaningfulness. According to Antonovsky (1987a, 1993), the three components are interrelated, and all of them are needed for successful coping. Comprehensibility is the cognitive component that deals with understanding what to do when facing stressful conditions. Manageability is the instrumental component that defines the ability to act in a certain stressful situation. Meaningfulness represents the motivational component and it refers to whether an individual feels that life makes sense, and whether at least some daily endeavours are worthwhile. According to the theory, meaningfulness is regarded as the most central component of sense of coherence, affecting both comprehensibility and manageability (Antonovsky, 1987a, 1993). The individual who scores high in all three of the components is considered to have a strong sense of coherence, which has been linked to good health in previous research (Lundberg, 1997; Gilbar, 1998; Kivimäki et al, 2000; Nilsson et al, 2001; Suominen et al, 2001; Nakamura et al, 2003; Poppius et al, 2003; Surtees et al, 2003; von Bothmer and Fridlund, 2003; Chumbler et al, 2004; Sjostrom et al, 2004; Tak-Ying Shiu, 2004; Lindfors et al, 2005; Savolainen et al, 2005).

Sense of coherence is hypothesised to be a fairly stable dispositional orientation of personality (Antonovsky et al, 1990; Sagy et al, 1990), which is founded on experiences in childhood and adolescence. An individual's sense of coherence is assumed to be fully developed and stabilised around the age of 30. Even if sense of coherence is said to be relatively stable in adulthood, this does not exclude the possibility that some variation in the strength of sense of coherence may occur during the life course. Major life events, for example, radical changes in working conditions, may affect an individual's general resistance resources and thus substantially change the strength of sense of coherence, even in older individuals (Antonovsky, 1987a, 1987b, 1991).

Sense of coherence and work stress

Most of the existing research on sense of coherence has been carried out into life stress circumstances. Sense of coherence has been employed less frequently in occupational stress research. Previous research has focused almost exclusively on psychosocial work stress exposures in relation to sense of coherence (Kalimo and Vuori, 1990; Ryland and Greenfeld, 1991; Feldt, 1997, 2000; Feldt et al, 2000a; Söderfeldt et al, 2000; Albertsen et al, 2001; Kalimo et al, 2002, 2003; Agardh et al, 2003; Nasermoaddeli et al, 2003; Hoge and Bussing, 2004), leaving the relationship between physical work stress exposures and sense of coherence less explored (Feldt, 1997; Kalimo et al, 2002, 2003). Sense of coherence was found to moderate the effect of adverse physical factors (such as poor lighting or soundproofing, dirt and dust, noise, crowded working space) on emotional exhaustion (Feldt, 1997). To my knowledge, studies combining physical demands and sense of coherence using a representative population sample have not been conducted.

The main, mediating, and moderating effects of sense of coherence on the association between psychosocial work environment and health have been investigated previously (Feldt, 1997; Feldt et al, 2000a; Albertsen et al, 2001). The main effect of sense of coherence on health has received strong support. People with a strong sense of coherence experience fewer work-related health complaints. There is also evidence that sense of coherence partly explains the relationship between adverse work exposure and stress symptoms (Feldt et al, 2000a; Albertsen et al, 2001). Regarding the moderating role of sense of coherence, there is some support for suggesting that people with a strong sense of coherence cope more efficiently with an adverse work environment than people with a weak sense of coherence (Feldt, 1997; Albertsen et al, 2001).

Two Swedish studies have previously explored the combination of the demand-control model and sense of coherence (Söderfeldt et al, 2000; Agardh et al, 2003). In the latter study, sense of coherence was gauged by the same three-item measure of the present study. The results of this case control study, based on a sample (*n*=4,821) of Swedish women residing in Stockholm, showed that low decision latitude in combination with low sense of coherence increased the risk of type 2 diabetes (Agardh et al, 2003). Based on a small sample of civil servants (*n*=103), the combination of emotional job strain and low sense of coherence increased the risk of emotional exhaustion and depersonalisation, respectively (Söderfeldt et al, 2000).

Material and methods

Study sample

The analyses in this chapter are based on the panel of the LNU surveys for 1991 and 2000. A cohort of employed Swedish men and women, 18-55 years old at baseline (1991), was followed for nine years. Physical and psychosocial work stress exposure and sense of coherence were measured at baseline (1991), and cumulative incidence (henceforth incidence) of psychological distress or musculoskeletal pain was predicted at follow-up (2000). Self-employed individuals and farmers were excluded from the cohort since one of the questions on decision latitude did not apply to them. The age span of 18-55 years was selected so that the individuals of the cohort could be potentially employed both in 1991 and 2000. All of them were gainfully employed in 1991, and worked at least 20 hours weekly. This gave a sample of 2,373 individuals (49.7% men, 50.3% women). In 2000 some of them (*n*=435, 50.1% men, 49.9% women) were no longer employed (possibly unemployed, on disability pension or self-employed), and some worked less than 20 hours weekly (*n*=25, 20% men, 80% women). The non-response rate of this age span (18-55 years) was 19.4% in 1991. Among those who responded in 1991 (3,906 individuals), 18% dropped out at follow-up in 2000.

Dependent variables

Two health outcomes were studied: psychological distress and musculoskeletal pain. The measure of psychological distress was based on an additive index answering the question: 'Have you had any of the following illnesses or ailments during the past 12 months: tiredness, sleeping disturbances, nervousness (anxiety, worry), depression, dejection, overexertion or psychiatric illness?'. To each item, the respondent was asked to answer 'No', 'Yes, mild' or 'Yes, severe'. Those subjects reporting at least one severe or three mild conditions for the first six items, or reporting mild or severe psychiatric illness, were categorised as having psychological distress.

Similarly, the measure of musculoskeletal pain was based on an additive index answering the question: 'Have you had any of the following illnesses or ailments during the past 12 months: pain in shoulders, back pain or sciatica, pain in hands, elbows, feet or knees?'. Those subjects reporting at least one severe or three mild conditions were categorised as having musculoskeletal pain.

Independent variables

Physical demands were measured by an additive index consisting of four items: 'Is your job physically demanding?'; 'Do you have to be able to lift 60kg in order to do your job?'; 'Does your job cause you to sweat on a daily basis?'; 'Does your job oblige you to adopt unsuitable work postures?'. Subjects answering 'Yes' were coded as being exposed to physical demands. Scores ranged from 0 to 4 and the index was dichotomised. Those with scores ≤2 were categorised as exposed to low physical demands (78%), and those with scores >2 as exposed to high physical demands (22%, approximately the most exposed quartile). Those with low physical demands at work were used as the reference group.

Psychosocial work stress was assessed by a measure for the demand–control model, in line with Karasek's initial operationalising of the model on the Swedish LNU surveys (see, for example, Karasek, 1979; Karasek et al, 1982). An identical measure has been employed in previous studies based on the same data material (le Grand et al, 2001). Two items measured psychological demands: 'Do you have to rush while working?'; 'Is your job psychologically demanding?'. Subjects answering 'Yes' to both questions were categorised as having high psychological demands. Similarly, decision latitude was captured by two questions: 'Can you decide your own pace of work?'; 'Is your job monotonous?'. Subjects answering 'No' to the first question and 'Yes' to the second question were categorised as having low control. The measures of psychological demands and decision latitude were then combined according to the demand–control model, giving four different work situations: active (high demands and high decision latitude), job strain (high demands and low decision latitude), passive (low demands and low decision latitude), and low strain (low demands and high decision latitude). In some analyses a dichotomous variable of the demand–control model was used comprising active, passive, and low strain situations contra job strain. Social support was not included in the analyses in this chapter since only one item on social support at work was available in the data.

Sense of coherence was gauged by a previously validated three-item measure (Lundberg and Nyström Peck, 1995). The three dimensions of the construct were assessed by one question each. Manageability: 'Do you usually see a solution to problems and difficulties that other people find hopeless?'. Meaningfulness: 'Do you usually feel that your daily life is a source of personal fulfilment?'. Comprehensibility: 'Do you usually feel that the things that happen to you in your daily life are hard to understand?'. The response alternatives were 'Yes, usually' (=2), 'Yes, sometimes' (=1), and 'No' (=0). The scoring was reversed for comprehensibility. Scores ranged from 0-6 and the index was split in line with previous studies (Lundberg, 1997), so that those with scores ≥4 were categorised as having a strong sense of coherence (83%) and those with scores <4 as having a weak sense of coherence (17%). Those with a strong sense of coherence were used as the reference group.

To assess the combinations of sense of coherence and physical demands and the demand-control model, respectively, two variables with four categories each were computed. First, the dichotomous variable of sense of coherence (strong versus weak) was combined with physical demands (low versus high) giving four categories: (1) strong sense of coherence and low physical demands; (2) strong sense of coherence and high physical demands; (3) weak sense of coherence and low physical demands; (4) weak sense of coherence and high physical demands. Second, sense of coherence was combined with the dichotomous variable of the demand-control model (job strain versus other job types). This gave a variable with four categories: (1) strong sense of coherence and no job strain; (2) strong sense of coherence and job strain; (3) weak sense of coherence and no job strain; (4) weak sense of coherence and job strain.

Age was divided into four groups: 18-25, 26-35, 36-45 and 46-55 years at baseline (1991), and 27-35, 36-45, 46-55 and 56-64 years at follow-up (2000). Those in the youngest age group were used as the reference group. To study whether the exposure time to noxious working conditions increased between 1991 and 2000, a dichotomous variable (working more than 40 hours per week versus working 40 hours or less per week) was computed.

Statistical analyses

All analyses were performed separately for men and women, and all multivariate analyses were adjusted for age at follow-up (2000). First, cross-tabulation analyses were performed to evaluate changes in work stress exposure, sense of coherence, and the two health outcomes in 1991 and 2000. Pearson chi-square tests were accomplished to evaluate whether gender differences in the frequencies were statistically significant.

Second, healthy individuals at baseline (1991) were selected to estimate the predictive role of work stress exposure and a weak sense of coherence on psychological distress or musculoskeletal pain incidence at follow-up. Work stress exposure and sense of coherence were measured at baseline. Multiple logistic regression analyses were applied to calculate odds ratios (OR) for the association between the exposure and the health outcomes. An OR of 1.0 indicates that work stress exposure or sense of coherence do not have an effect on the probability of psychological distress or musculoskeletal pain incidence. Thus, the reference groups were given the OR of 1.0, and OR greater than 1.0 stated the odds (or risk) of psychological distress or musculoskeletal pain incidence compared to the reference group. Ninety-five per cent confidence intervals were also calculated. When 1.0 is within the 95% confidence interval there is no significant risk for psychological distress or musculoskeletal pain incidence compared to the reference group (see Pagano and Gauvreau, 2000).

Third, the moderating effect of a strong sense of coherence on the two work stress exposures was investigated. A moderator is a variable that changes the direction or strength of the relationship between an independent and dependent variable. For instance, a dichotomous independent variable's effect on the dependent variable varies as a function of another dichotomous variable, that is, the moderator (see Baron and Kenny, 1986). Healthy individuals at baseline were selected; the interactions of sense of coherence and work stress exposure were measured at baseline, and psychological distress or musculoskeletal pain incidence were predicted at the nine-year follow-up. Odds ratios were calculated for the interaction effects of sense of coherence and the two work stress exposures, respectively, on newly reported psychological distress or musculoskeletal pain. Those with a strong sense of coherence and low work stress exposure were selected as the reference group. The analyses were performed using SPSS 12.0 software.

Results

Work stress, sense of coherence and the health outcomes

The distributions of included variables are described in Table 5.1. Since the data consisted of a prospective cohort, the individuals became nine years older during the study period. This is reflected in the distribution of the age groups; in 1991 the subjects were 18-55 years, and in 2000, consequently, 27-64 years. Also, some people were no longer employed in 2000. Therefore, the distributions of the work stress exposures in 2000 are calculated on the basis of those individuals who were still in work in 2000 (n=1,938).

Cross-tabulations showed that working conditions deteriorated for both men and women between the years 1991 and 2000, yet, the share of physical demands decreased for men by 3.3% between 1991 and 2000. Physical demands increased by 1.4% for women. Consequently, the gender difference in physical demands fell from 10% (1991) to 5.3% (2000), with men still the more exposed group. The share of low strain and passive jobs decreased. Active jobs and job strain increased, with a remarkable increase in job strain (5.6% for men and 5.4% for women). However, the share of job strain was approximately 11% higher among women than men at both measuring periods. In addition to deteriorating psychosocial working conditions, the exposure time to noxious conditions increased during the study period. The share of men and women working more than 40 hours per week increased notably (16.1% men, 12.9% women).

Sense of coherence remained reasonably stable among the subjects of this cohort. The share of those with a weak sense of coherence fell slightly among men (1.4%) and rose among women (2.1%) between 1991 and 2000. In this

Table 5.1: Distributions of independent and dependent variables: cohort of Swedish men and women employed in 1991 and 2000, χ^2-tests for gender differences

| | 1991 | | | | | 2000[a] | | | | |
| | Men | | Women | | | Men | | Women | | |
	n	%	*n*	%	χ^2	*n*	%	*n*	%	χ^2
Age group					ns					ns
18-25	182	15.4	187	15.7						
26-35	328	27.8	339	28.4		223	18.9	220	18.4	
36-45	363	30.8	371	31.1		327	27.7	335	27.9	
46-55	306	26.0	297	24.9		357	30.3	383	31.2	
56-64						272	23.1	256	22.3	
Physical demands					***					***
High	329	27.9	214	17.9		236	24.6	189	19.3	
Low	850	72.1	980	82.1		725	75.4	788	80.7	
Demand-control model					***					***
Job strain	131	11.1	263	22.0		161	16.7	268	27.4	
Passive	227	19.3	285	23.9		171	17.8	212	21.7	
Active	294	24.9	229	19.2		244	25.4	202	20.7	
Low strain	527	44.7	417	34.9		385	40.1	295	30.2	
Work intensity					***					***
>40 hours per week	347	29.4	162	13.6		434	45.5	254	26.5	
≤40 hours per week	832	70.6	1032	86.4		527	54.5	723	73.5	
Sense of coherence					***					ns
Weak	228	19.3	176	14.7		211	17.9	201	16.8	
Strong	951	80.7	1018	85.3		968	82.1	993	83.2	
Psychological distress					***					***
Yes	72	6.1	133	11.1		136	11.5	250	20.9	
No	1107	93.9	1061	88.9		1043	88.5	944	79.1	
Musculoskeletal pain					***					***
Yes	224	19.0	297	24.9		303	25.7	396	33.2	
No	955	81.0	897	75.1		876	74.3	798	66.8	
n	1,179	49.9	1,194	50.1		1,179	49.9	1,194	50.1	

*$p<0.05$, **$p<0.01$, ***$p<0.000$, ns = not significant

Notes: [a] In 2000 435 people were no longer employed. The distributions in 2000 of physical demands, demand-control model and work intensity include employed men (*n*=961) and women (*n*=977).

sample, fewer women had a weak sense of coherence than men in both 1991 and 2000, but this gender difference was lower in 2000. A more detailed mobility analysis of sense of coherence between the measuring periods (not reported here) showed that those with a strong sense of coherence in both 1991 and 2000 constituted the biggest group (70.3% of men, 74.8% of women), and those with a weak sense of coherence at both measuring periods constituted the smallest group (7.5% of men and 6.4% of women). The share of those whose sense of coherence improved from weak to strong was 11.8% in men and 8.4% in women. The share of those whose sense of coherence deteriorated from strong to weak was 10.3% in men and 10.5% in women.

The prevalence of psychological distress and musculoskeletal pain increased in both men and women between 1991 and 2000. The prevalence of psychological distress was lower for men than for women at both measuring periods. Psychological distress increased by 5.4% among men, and 9.8% among women. Thus, the gender difference in psychological distress also rose from 5% (1991) to 9.4% (2000). Similarly, the prevalence of musculoskeletal pain was lower among men than among women at both measuring periods. Musculoskeletal pain increased by 6.7% for men and 8.3% for women. The gender difference also increased for this health impairment during the study period (from 5.9% to 7.5%). However, it should be borne in mind that the respondents aged nine years during the study period, and this is reflected in the prevalence of ill health.

Predictive role of work stress and sense of coherence

Among men, high physical demands predicted new cases of psychological distress (OR 2.24) compared to those with low physical demands (Table 5.2(a), model 1). Job strain (OR 2.59), passive job (OR 1.87), and active job (OR 1.69, barely significant) increased the odds for psychological distress incidence compared to those with a low strain job (Table 5.2(a), model 2). A weak sense of coherence did not predict psychological distress incidence in men (Table 5.2(a), model 3). The full model showed that high physical demands (OR 2.33), job strain (OR 2.64), and active job (OR 1.91) predicted new cases of psychological distress in men compared to reference categories (Table 5.2(a), model 4).

In women, high physical demands did not predict new cases of psychological distress (Table 5.2(b), model 1). Although the demand-control indicator does not reach statistical significance, job strain (OR 1.56) increased the odds for psychological distress incidence compared to those with a low strain job (Table 5.2(b), model 2). Having a weak sense of coherence doubled the odds for psychological distress incidence (OR 2.19) compared to those with a strong sense of coherence (Table 5.2(b), model 3). These associations remained relatively unaffected in the fully adjusted model 4 (Table 5.2(b)).

In men, high physical demands (OR 2.14) predicted new cases of musculoskeletal pain (Table 5.3(a), model 1). Psychosocial work stress also predicted musculoskeletal pain incidence; active job (OR 1.50), job strain (OR 1.77) and passive job (OR 1.54). However, the estimates of these job categories were of similar magnitude (Table 5.3(a), model 2). Sense of coherence (OR 1.66) significantly increased the odds of musculoskeletal pain incidence in men (Table 5.3(a), model 3). In the full model the effects of high physical demands (OR 2.20) and active job (OR 1.74) strengthened, while the effects of job strain (OR 1.70), passive job (OR 1.44), and a weak sense of coherence (OR 1.60) attenuated (Table 5.3(a), model 4).

The case for women was similar: high physical demands (OR 1.98) predicted musculoskeletal pain incidence (Table 5.3(b), model 1). Job strain (OR 1.80) and passive jobs (OR 1.71) increased the odds of musculoskeletal pain incidence

Table 5.2: Odds ratios (OR) for psychological distress in 2000 by work stress exposures and sense of coherence in 1991: men and women employed in 1991

	Model 1	Model 2	Model 3	Model 4
	OR (95% CI)	OR (95% CI)	OR (95% CI)	OR (95% CI)
(a) Men employed in 1991[a]				
Physical demands	***			***
High	2.24 (1.47-3.42)			2.33 (1.51-3.59)
Low	1.00			1.00
Demand-control model		*		*
Job strain		2.59 (1.39-4.81)		2.64 (1.41-4.94)
Passive		1.87 (1.07-3.25)		1.74 (0.99-3.05)
Active		1.69 (0.99-2.88)		1.91 (1.11-3.27)
Low strain		1.00		1.00
Sense of coherence			ns	ns
Weak			1.06 (0.63-1.78)	0.97 (0.57-1.65)
Strong			1.00	1.00
n	1,107	1,107	1,107	1,107
(b) Women employed in 1991[a]				
Physical demands	ns			ns
High	1.02 (0.66-1.55)			0.88 (0.57-1.36)
Low	1.00			1.00
Demand-control model		ns		ns
Job strain		1.56 (1.02-2.41)		1.55 (1.00-2.41)
Passive		1.13 (0.73-1.74)		1.09 (0.70-1.68)
Active		0.99 (0.62-1.59)		1.00 (0.62-1.61)
Low strain		1.00		1.00
Sense of coherence			***	***
Weak			2.19 (1.45-3.30)	2.18 (1.43-3.30)
Strong			1.00	1.00
n	1,061	1,061	1,061	1,061

Note: [a] All models adjusted for age.

*p<0.05, **p<0.01, ***p<0.000, ns = not significant

(Table 5.3(b), model 2). In women, sense of coherence (OR 1.50) predicted musculoskeletal pain incidence in a similar manner as in men. However, in women the OR was not significantly different from the reference category. In the full model, the significant effects of high physical demands, job strain and passive job on musculoskeletal pain incidence decreased (Table 5.3(b), model 4).

Moderating role of sense of coherence

Men with a weak sense of coherence and high physical demands had a higher odds (OR 2.40) of psychological distress incidence than men with a strong sense of coherence and low physical demands. Men with a strong sense of

Table 5.3: Odds ratios (OR) for musculoskeletal pain in 2000 by work stress exposures and sense of coherence in 1991: men and women employed in 1991

	Model 1	Model 2	Model 3	Model 4
	OR (95% CI)	OR (95% CI)	OR (95% CI)	OR (95% CI)
(a) Men employed in 1991[a]				
Physical demands	***			***
High	2.14 (1.50-3.05)			2.20 (1.52-3.16)
Low	1.00			1.00
Demand-control model		*		*
Job strain		1.77 (1.05-2.99)		1.70 (1.00-2.90)
Passive		1.54 (1.00-2.37)		1.44 (0.93-2.24)
Active		1.50 (1.02-2.23)		1.74 (1.16-2.61)
Low strain		1.00		1.00
Sense of coherence			**	*
Weak			1.66 (1.14-2.42)	1.60 (1.08-2.35)
Strong			1.00	1.00
n	955	955	955	955
(b) Women employed in 1991[a]				
Physical demands	**			*
High	1.81 (1.20-2.74)			1.62 (1.06-2.47)
Low	1.00			1.00
Demand-control model		*		*
Job strain		1.80 (1.18-2.74)		1.62 (1.06-2.50)
Passive		1.71 (1.12-2.59)		1.63 (1.07-2.49)
Active		1.08 (0.68-1.73)		1.06 (0.66-1.69)
Low strain		1.00		1.00
Sense of coherence			ns	ns
Weak			1.50 (0.96-2.32)	1.34 (0.86-2.11)
Strong			1.00	1.00
n	897	897	897	897

Note: [a] All models adjusted for age.

*p<0.05, **p<0.01, ***p<0.000, ns = not significant

coherence and high physical demands also had higher odds (OR 2.12) of psychological distress incidence than men with a strong sense of coherence and low physical demands. The OR decreased slightly from 2.40 to 2.12 depending on the strength of sense of coherence in the categories exposed to high physical demands (Table 5.4(a)).

Women with a weak sense of coherence and high physical demands had higher odds (OR 2.18) of psychological distress incidence than women with a strong sense of coherence and low physical demands. A strong sense of coherence and high physical demands (OR 0.92) was not significantly different from the reference category. When men and women were studied together, there was a similar trend. A weak sense of coherence and high physical demands (OR 1.93), and a strong sense of coherence and high physical demands (OR 1.27, not significant) gave higher odds of psychological distress incidence than did the combination of a strong sense of coherence and low physical demands. Thus, there is some evidence that a strong sense of coherence may moderate the adverse effect of high physical demands on psychological distress incidence (Table 5.4(a)).

The trend for the combined effect of sense of coherence and physical demands on musculoskeletal pain incidence was similar for men and women, and also when men and women were studied together (Table 5.4(a)). The effects were, however, stronger for men than women. When men and women were studied together, having a weak sense of coherence and high physical demands (OR 3.05) increased the odds of musculoskeletal pain incidence threefold compared to those with a strong sense of coherence and low physical demands. A strong sense of coherence reduced this OR; the combination of a strong sense of coherence and high physical demands generated an OR of 1.81 of musculoskeletal pain incidence. Thus, a strong sense of coherence moderated the adverse effect of high physical demands on musculoskeletal pain incidence both in men and women (Table 5.4(a)).

In men, the combined effect of sense of coherence and job strain on psychological distress incidence was not significant (Table 5.4(b)). Women, with a weak sense of coherence and job strain, had a higher odds (OR 2.39) of psychological distress incidence than women with a strong sense of coherence and no physical demands. Women with a strong sense of coherence and job strain also had a higher odds (OR 1.64) of psychological distress incidence than women with a strong sense of coherence and no physical demands. A strong sense of coherence thus modified the adverse effect of job strain on psychological distress incidence in women. However, the combination of a weak sense of coherence and other job types of the demand–control model also created excess odds (OR 2.45) of psychological distress in women. Yet, it should be kept in mind from the preceding analyses (Table 5.2) that a weak sense of coherence predicted psychological distress incidence in women, but not in men.

When men and women were studied together, those with a weak sense of coherence and job strain (OR 2.24) had higher odds of psychological distress incidence than those with a strong sense of coherence and low physical demands. A strong sense of coherence and job strain (OR 1.85) also increased the odds of psychological distress incidence, but to a lesser extent. Thus, there is some evidence that a strong sense of coherence moderates the adverse effect of job strain on psychological distress incidence when men and women are studied together, and in women only (Table 54(b)).

The combined effect of sense of coherence and job strain on musculoskeletal pain incidence was not significant for men or for women (Table 5.4(b)). However, when men and women were studied together, the effect modification was significant. Those with a weak sense of coherence and job strain had higher odds (OR 1.84) of musculoskeletal pain incidence than those with a strong sense of coherence and no job strain. Those with a strong sense of coherence and job

Table 5.4(a): Odds ratios (OR) for psychological distress and musculoskeletal pain in 2000 by combination of sense of coherence and physical demands in 1991: men and women employed in 1991[a]

	Psychological distress			Musculoskeletal pain		
	Men	Women	All	Men	Women	All
	OR (95 % CI)	OR (95 % CI)	OR (95 % CI)	OR (95 % CI)	OR (95 % CI)	OR (95 % CI)
SOC/physical demands	**	**	*	***	**	***
Strong SOC/low demands	1.00	1.00	1.00	1.00	1.00	1.00
Weak SOC/low demands	0.84 (0.39-1.83)	2.15 (1.24-3.75)	1.45 (0.98-2.14)	1.51 (0.94-2.45)	1.34 (0.79-2.25)	1.38 (0.97-1.97)
Strong SOC/high demands	2.12 (1.33-3.40)	0.92 (0.52-1.71)	1.27 (0.92-1.77)	2.03 (1.35-3.05)	1.68 (1.05-2.68)	1.81 (1.34-2.46)
Weak SOC/high demands	2.40 (1.20-4.83)	2.18 (1.05-4.54)	1.93 (1.18-3.17)	3.43 (1.90-6.18)	2.78 (1.25-6.15)	3.05 (1.91-4.87)
n	1.107	1.061	2.168	955	897	1.852

Note: [a] All models adjusted for age.; *p<0.05, **p<0.01, ***p<0.000, ns = not significant; SOC = sense of coherence

Table 5.4(b): Odds ratios (OR) for psychological distress and musculoskeletal pain in 2000 by combination of sense of coherence and job strain in 1991: men and women employed in 1991[a]

	Psychological distress			Musculoskeletal pain		
	Men	Women	All	Men	Women	All
	OR (95 % CI)	OR (95 % CI)	OR (95 % CI)	OR (95 % CI)	OR (95 % CI)	OR (95 % CI)
SOC/job strain	ns	***	***	ns	ns	**
Strong SOC/others	1.00	1.00	1.00	1.00	1.00	1.00
Weak SOC/ others	1.05 (0.59-1.86)	2.45 (1.53-3.91)	1.58 (1.11-2.25)	1.70 (1.13-2.54)	1.60 (0.96-2.68)	1.65 (1.20-2.26)
Strong SOC/job strain	1.88 (1.01-3.51)	1.64 (1.08-2.49)	1.85 (1.31-2.62)	1.47 (0.83-2.59)	1.55 (1.04-2.30)	1.58 (1.15-2.17)
Weak SOC/ job strain	1.91 (0.64-5.74)	2.39 (1.07-5.36)	2.24 (1.18-4.25)	1.94 (0.78-4.83)	1.78 (0.79-4.00)	1.84 (1.01-3.37)
n	1,107	1,061	2,168	955	897	1.852

Note: [a] All models adjusted for age.; *p<0.05, **p<0.01, ***p<0.000, ns = not significant; SOC = sense of coherence

strain also had higher odds (OR 1.58) of musculoskeletal pain incidence than those with a strong sense of coherence and no job strain. Yet, the difference between these OR was not very substantial. Thus, this result indicates that a strong sense of coherence only slightly modifies the effect of job strain on musculoskeletal pain incidence among employed men and women in Sweden (Table 5.4(b)).

Discussion

This study, which focused on the 1990s, was based on a prospective population-based cohort of gainfully employed men and women in Sweden. It elucidated gender differences and changes in physical and psychosocial work stress exposure, sense of coherence and prevalence of psychological distress and musculoskeletal pain in 1991 and 2000. The predictive role of work stress exposure and sense of coherence on psychological distress or musculoskeletal pain was explored. Finally, the moderating role of sense of coherence on the effect of work stress on psychological distress or musculoskeletal pain was investigated.

Changes during the study period

In line with previous research (le Grand et al, 2001; Rostila, 2004), cross-tabulations also showed that psychosocial working conditions deteriorated between 1991 and 2000 for the cohort of the present study. Small changes were observed for physical demands; a fall (3.8%) in high physical demands among men, and a slight rise (1.4%) in high physical demands among women. According to a previous study, fewer men than women are still employed in physically demanding jobs at older age, and the high physical workload among women in the social and health care sector is likely to contribute to the gender differences in health (Aittomäki et al, 2005). The cohort of the present study aged by nine years during the study period. It is plausible that the changes in the proportions of high physical demands reflect that it is more common for women than men to still have physically demanding work at older age. Taken as a whole, the deterioration in working conditions during the study period was worse for women than men (see also Chapter Three).

The stability of sense of coherence has been questioned and caution has been advised when using sense of coherence to represent a stable global orientation (Smith et al, 2003). However, in line with theory (Antonovsky, 1987a, 1991, 1993) and previous investigations (Feldt et al, 2000b; Kivimäki et al, 2000), sense of coherence remained moderately stable among the subjects of this panel sample. There was a significant gender difference in sense of coherence at baseline, showing that women were more likely to have a strong sense of coherence than men; but with increasing age this difference weakened, and it was no longer significant at follow-up. The majority of men (77.8%) and women (81.2%) had a stable sense of coherence between 1991 and 2000. Hence, these results indicate that sense of coherence represents a stable disposition of personality (Antonovsky et al, 1990; Sagy et al, 1990). However, a more detailed analysis of the stability of sense of coherence in this cohort should be conducted in order to fully confirm Antonovsky's hypothesis of a stable disposition of personality, but a detailed stability analysis of sense of coherence was outside the frame of the present study.

Work stress and sense of coherence as predictors of ill health

High physical demands, job strain and active job predicted psychological distress incidence in men, and job strain predicted psychological distress incidence in women. Previous findings suggest that psychosocial work exposures may be more significant determinants of psychological wellbeing in male workers than in female workers (Vermeulen and Mustard, 2000).

High physical demands predicted musculoskeletal pain incidence in both men and women, thus confirming earlier findings (Punnett and Wegman, 2004). Psychosocial work stress, in terms of active job and job strain in men, and passive job and job strain in women, also predicted musculoskeletal pain incidence. According to previous findings, job strain predicts back and neck injuries (Rugulies and Krause, 2005). A positive relationship was found between upper extremity problems or neck pain, and high psychological demands or low control at work (Ariëns et al, 2001; Bongers et al, 2002). In the present study, psychological demands and job control were combined in line with the demand-control model (Karasek and Theorell, 1990). The results suggest that there may be a gender difference in the associations between the different aspects of the demand-control model and musculoskeletal pain. It may be that the demand aspect of the demand-control model is associated with musculoskeletal pain in men, and the control aspect in women.

When the predictive role of sense of coherence was studied, the analyses focused on whether a weak sense of coherence was a predictor of psychological distress or musculoskeletal pain, rather than the health-promoting role of a strong sense of coherence. A previous study chose a similar approach and claimed that the results may be reversed: not having a weak sense of coherence increases the possibility of being healthy (Lundberg and Nyström Peck, 1994). Similarly, the status of sense of coherence as a salutary phenomenon that is distinguishable from pathogenic determinants of health has been questioned, since a weak sense of coherence was found to predict adverse health prospects more than a strong sense of coherence predicted good health (Kivimäki et al, 2000). Not many studies have reported gender differences in the relationship between sense of coherence and health. In the present study, the expected predictive effect of a weak sense of coherence on psychological distress was found for women. No predictive association was observed between a weak sense of coherence and psychological distress in men. These results are in line with previous findings (Kivimäki et al, 2000). A predictive association between a weak sense of coherence and musculoskeletal pain was found in men. A similar association was found in women, but the estimate was barely significant (OR 1.50 [0.96-2.32]). Whether a weak sense of coherence can be regarded as a determinant of ill health in a sample of gainfully employed men and women depends evidently on gender and the specific health outcome in question.

Sense of coherence as a moderator

The moderating role of sense of coherence seemed to depend on gender, work stress exposure and health outcome. The most substantial moderating effects can be summarised as follows: (1) a strong sense of coherence moderated the adverse effects of physical demands on musculoskeletal pain incidence in men and in women; and (2) a strong sense of coherence moderated the adverse effects of job strain on psychological distress incidence in women, and when men and women were studied together, but not in men. In line with the theoretical argumentation of sense of coherence (Antonovsky, 1979, 1987a), viewing life as comprehensible, manageable and meaningful apparently provided employed men and women with the strength to better meet challenges in the workplace.

However, it should be noted that even if a strong sense of coherence moderated the adverse effects of work stress in some cases, those individuals with a strong sense of coherence and adverse work stress exposure also had an increased risk of ill health. It can be argued that there is no such thing as resistance power against work stress; sooner or later everyone will be affected by adverse working conditions, even if one has a buffering personality disposition. "Everyone will boil, but at different temperatures", to quote Professor emeritus Lennart Levi (personal communication, 2002). The main focus of work-related stress research should therefore be on working conditions and not on the procedures for managing stress (Antonovsky, 1987b).

Gender differences

According to previous findings, there are real differences in the factors that predict women's and men's health (see, for example, Denton and Walters, 1999). The results of the present study revealed gender differences in the ability of work stress exposures and sense of coherence to predict health outcomes. Both physical and psychosocial exposure at work significantly increased the risk of psychological distress in men, and to a lesser extent also in women (job strain only). However, a weak sense of coherence increased the risk of future psychological distress more than twofold in women, while it had no effect in men. This could indicate that viewing the world as comprehensible, manageable and meaningful is more important for women's psychological wellbeing than men's. In other words, women's worlds may be more complex than men's, since women more often than men have to divide themselves between home duties and work–life challenges. According to a Swedish study, employed women's health was determined by the interaction between conditions at work and household duties, whereas men responded more selectively to long working hours (Krantz et al, 2005). Thus, it might be the case that strengthening women's sense of coherence in both private and working life spheres, and facilitating the balance of these spheres, could promote psychological wellbeing in women. It should be borne in mind, however, that the women in the present study at both measuring times had a slightly greater share of strong sense of coherence than men. Consequently, because of this gender difference in the predictive role of sense of coherence for psychological distress, the findings about the moderating role of sense of coherence for the impact of job strain on psychological distress also need to be interpreted carefully.

Regarding musculoskeletal pain, the results were more or less similar in men and in women. Still, it should be noted that active jobs for men, and passive jobs for women seem to be as harmful as job strain for the risk of musculoskeletal pain. Even if similar numbers of women and men are in gainful employment in Sweden, they tend to have different kinds of jobs, which indicate that the Swedish labour market is segregated by gender (Nermo, 1999). There are also big gender differences in part-time working and in the reasons for working part time (Evertsson, 2004). These factors probably also contribute to the gender differences in ill health found in the present study.

Conclusion

The strength of the present study is in its longitudinal design, and that the analyses are based on a representative population sample of employed men and women in Sweden. Following a cohort over time is advantageous for establishing the causal direction between exposures and outcomes. Also, results are generalisable when one uses a representative population sample rather than samples based on specific occupational groups.

There are nevertheless some limitations in the present study. First, sense of coherence was gauged by a simplified three-item measure designed for survey questionnaires addressed to population samples. However, a validation study of the three-item measure showed acceptable correspondence with Antonovsky's original instrument (Lundberg and Nyström Peck, 1995). The same three-item measure of sense of coherence used in the present study has also been employed in previous studies (Agardh et al, 2003; Surtees et al, 2003; Lindfors et al, 2005). Second, the index of physical demands was dichotomised in order to be more comparable with the dichotomous demand-control model in the analyses of the moderating role of sense of coherence. The continuous scale of physical demands was initially analysed in relation to psychological distress and musculoskeletal pain. Since those with many physical exposures seemed to have the highest risk of ill health, the index was split so that those with two or less exposures were categorised as having low physical demands, and those with three to four exposures were categorised as having high physical demands. The associations between physical work exposures and health outcomes are typically non-linear, with those with a large number of exposures being very much more likely to have less than good health (see Chapter Three). Third, it can be argued that the combined effects of work stress exposure and sense of coherence should have been assessed by measures commonly used for testing biological interaction, for example (1) the relative excess risk due to interaction, (2) the attributable proportion due to interaction, or (3) the synergy index (Rothman, 2002; Ahlbom and Alfredsson, 2005; Andersson et al, 2005). These measures were in fact estimated according to recommended instructions (Lundberg et al, 1996; Andersson et al, 2005). Yet, it is difficult to get significant estimates for biological interaction in relatively small samples representative of the population. The group exposed to one of the adverse work stress exposures and also having a weak sense of coherence was smallest (2.9-4.5%), which most likely contributed to insignificant estimates. Nevertheless, the estimate for synergy index for high physical demands and weak sense of coherence in relation to pain (SI 1.70 [CI 0.73-3.94]), and to psychological distress (SI 1.26 [CI 0.41-3.81]) suggests that there does exist a biological interaction between high physical demands and weak sense of coherence, even if the estimates were not statistically significant. In the case of job strain and weak sense of coherence, the estimates for the synergy index <1 suggested that there is no biological interaction between these factors.

Despite these limitations, the results of the present study indicate that a strong sense of coherence moderated the work stress effect on health in specific situations. Substantial gender differences were revealed in the associations between work stress exposures, sense of coherence and health. The moderating role of sense of coherence also varied according to these factors. Thus, in future studies on work stress, sense of coherence and health, men and women should be studied separately.

SIX

Psychosocial work environment and stress-related health complaints: an analysis of children's and adolescents' situation in school

Bitte Modin and Viveca Östberg

Introduction

In the broad perspective applied in Nordic welfare research, Swedish children and adolescents are generally well off. The majority are rich in material resources, have a high housing standard, are seldom subject to threatening events, do not have problems with schoolwork and have good relations with parents as well as peers (Jonsson and Östberg, 2001). The fact that problems in these areas are quite uncommon does, of course, not make the situation of the exposed groups less important. Furthermore, there is one area in which problems appear to be rather common. Several studies have shown that psychological health problems and psychosomatic complaints are frequent and more common today than one or two decades ago (Danielson, 2003; Berntsson and Köhler, 2001; see also Jonsson and Östberg, 2001). High levels of these types of complaint are not unique to Sweden; they exist in several other European countries (Currie et al, 2000; Haugland et al, 2001). It is worth aiming for a better understanding of these health problems and their causes; the Swedish government has now put forward psychological health problems among children as a public health issue that should be given special attention (Proposition, 2002).

Social class is generally a good point of departure in the search for causes of health problems and when our aim is to understand how society affects the health of its citizens (Marmot et al, 1987). Societal groupings typically involve differences in living conditions that may result in health disparities (Marmot, 2004). With regard to the psychological health of young people, however, social class differences have been shown to be small or non-existent (West, 1997; West and Sweeting, 2003). This is true also for Sweden (Östberg et al, 2006). Consequently, the living conditions of importance to these health problems are not closely connected to social class.

Psychological health problems and somatic complaints are, to some extent, believed to be stress-related (Natvig et al, 1999; Bovier et al, 2004), and one reason behind their increase may be a general intensification of stress in children's and adolescents' day-to-day life (Danielson and Marklund, 2000; NBHW, 2001; Torsheim and Wold, 2001a). It has been claimed that school, that is, children's work environment, is one arena where conditions can cause stress among children (CO, 2004:03).

The importance of conditions at work for the adult population has been commonly acknowledged, with much attention paid to the links between the psychosocial work environment, stress and health. The demand-control-support model represents a frequently used line of thinking (Karasek, 1979; Johnson, 1986; Karasek and Theorell, 1990). At special risk of stress-related ill health are those with high demands, low control and a low degree of social support.

It is uncommon to view pupils' situation in school as a work environment with a potential influence on health. In Sweden, the compulsory school comprises all children aged 7-16, the vast majority of whom then continue their education in upper secondary school. Pupils normally spend five days a week and about 40 weeks a year in school. This makes conditions in school an important dimension of young people's welfare.

Using the demand-control-support model as the frame of reference and self-reported data from a nationally representative sample of Swedish compulsory school pupils, this chapter investigates stress-related aspects of health, namely psychosomatic complaints and psychological wellbeing. The links between the welfare state and the school, and between the work environment and health, will be discussed and the purpose of the study more thoroughly outlined below.

Welfare state and the school

The Swedish Education Act of 1985 states that all children and youths are entitled to equal education irrespective of gender, place of residence and social or economic factors. In line with this, all education in the public school system is free of charge and there are usually no costs for teaching materials, school meals, health services or transport. Most children and adolescents attend a compulsory school that is run by the municipality and located in the neighborhood. The parents are free, however, to choose another municipal or privately run school. The share of students attending the latter type of school in 2004 was 6.2% (CO, 2004:06). Both privately run and municipal schools are obliged to work to certain basic objectives and must be approved and evaluated by the National Agency for Education.

The relevance of the economy for schools as a whole became highly visible during the Swedish economic recession of the 1990s (Palme et al, 2003). As a joint consequence of the recession and demographic changes, the number of compulsory schoolteachers per 100 pupils fell from 9.4 in 1991 to 7.6 in 1999 (NAE, 2001), and this level remains practically unchanged today. Moreover, the proportion of teachers with university-level training has fallen. It does, however, vary considerably, now ranging from 56% to 98% between different municipalities (NAE, 2003).

The situation of children and adolescents in school can be seen as analogous to the work environment for adults. Since 1990, the Swedish Work Environment Act also covers schools. This means that school principals, like employers, are responsible for organising work in a way that promotes health among pupils. However, an obvious difference between adult workplaces and schools is that the latter can be regarded as more homogeneous. Many aspects of the physical environment, the setting and schoolwork are similar for all pupils. However, a closer scrutiny of the school environment reveals differences between schools and school classes. These differences may stem from various factors, such as the municipality's financial situation and priorities, individual principals and teachers, as well as the composition of students in terms of ethnicity and social class.

Work environment and health

A large amount of empirical evidence suggests that stressful working conditions have detrimental effects on adult health. While demands are a natural part of working life, a disproportionate level of stress-inducing requirements and obligations may, in the long run, endanger an individual's wellbeing. This is especially true for those who lack the means to deal with such stressful situations, for example if one has a low level of control. In empirical studies, demanding working conditions usually refer to time pressure, work pace, workload and conflicting demands. An individual's degree of control over his/her working conditions, on the other hand, depends on the degree of task variety (or skill discretion) and the autonomy (or decision authority) that the job offers. Put differently, it refers to "the worker's ability to control his or her own activities and skill usage" (Karasek and Theorell, 1990, p 60).

By combining these two aspects of working conditions, four different types of jobs may be discerned, each of which reflects a specific kind of psychosocial work environment (see Figure 6.1). The 'low strain job' has low demands and high control. These jobs are characterised by relaxed and leisurely working conditions. Although they may offer few challenges, the possibility of responding to every demand optimally makes this group of employees less vulnerable to stress-related illness. The 'active job' is highly demanding, but also offers a high degree of control. Provided that the level of demand is not overwhelming, these working conditions tend to cause a positive spiral of job-induced learning through which the worker develops new coping strategies that may prevent stress and promote self-esteem. The 'passive job', in which both demands and control are low, gives rise to a reverse state of affairs. Despite the fact that these working conditions are demotivating, the low level of demands still puts the passive jobholders at about the same risk as the active jobholders when it comes to stress-induced illness, according to the originators of the model.

Figure 6.1: The demand–control–support model

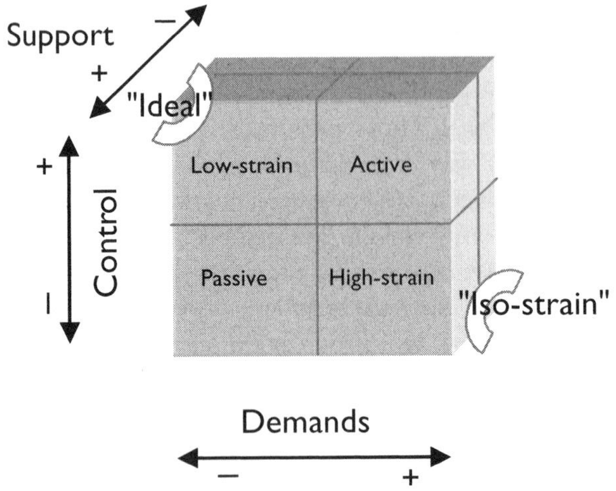

Sources: Karasek and Theorell (1990); Theorell (2003)

Finally, the 'high strain job' is defined by the combination of high demands and low control and is the unhealthiest of the four working conditions presented so far. A heavy workload in combination with insufficient freedom of action to cope with the situation is typical for these kinds of jobs. Here, energy from stimulation followed by constraints on the worker's optimal response generates unused residual strain that, in the long run, may cause feelings of hopelessness and stress-related illness.

There is also a third dimension to the psychosocial work environment, namely social support (Johnson, 1986). The buffering effects of social support against stress and disease have been widely acknowledged (Cassel, 1976; Berkman and Syme, 1979; Broadhead et al, 1983; Cohen and Syme, 1985; Berkman et al, 2000; Cohen et al, 2000). Important sources of social support in the psychosocial work environment are emotional and instrumental support (Karasek and Theorell, 1990). The former refers to the integration and trust between co-workers and supervisors, while the latter concerns assistance and guidance by co-workers or supervisors that may facilitate certain work tasks. Adding this third dimension to the model doubles the number of job types, the two extremes being the 'ideal' versus the 'iso-strained' psychosocial work environment. While the 'ideal' working conditions offer a high degree of control in combination with low job demands and a high level of social support, the 'iso-strained' job is the direct opposite, involving a considerably increased risk of stress-related illness (Theorell, 2003).

Applying demand, control and support to schoolchildren

It may well prove fruitful to view and analyse the psychosocial work environment of schoolchildren in the same way as we do with adults. However, there are several ways in which the situation of schoolchildren differs from that of the adult working population, and these need to be clarified. An important aspect of adults' ability to control their work has been labelled task variety (or skill discretion). This focuses, among other things, on the degree to which the job involves learning new things and developing new skills – something that would seem highly applicable to school pupils. Another aspect of control is autonomy, something that we may assume to be less applicable to pupils. Children are not always seen as actors who benefit from having the kind of own resources that make decisions and action possible. Autonomous decision making for pupils is a stated goal of the Swedish school curriculum, although pupils themselves maintain that their influence in school is quite limited (NAE, 2004a). In addition, the aim of schoolwork, even though it may be carried out in a variety of ways, is all-embracing, which means that certain aspects of objective demands are highly standardised. One general demand, for example, is to meet the basic standards set for each educational level.

These differences between pupils and employed adults imply that the working conditions of schoolchildren are more homogeneous than those of the adult working population, both when it comes to objective demands and scope of control. Although the spectrum of demands and control is narrower for pupils than for adult jobholders, the health-related implications of the joint effects of these two dimensions need not necessarily be any less. Previous studies have shown that the model holds within more homogeneous groups of occupations (Turner, 1980; Wahlstedt, 2001; Muhonen and Torkelson, 2003). With regard to social support, however, there is no reason to believe that the variation should be smaller among pupils than employees. Pupils report a considerable variation in the degree to which they receive help from teachers, receive emotional support from other pupils and experience conflicts with both teachers and classmates (Östberg, 2001b). The school setting is a social arena in which social relations, including peer status, are of consequence for an individual's identity and self-esteem. Studies show that these factors are related to the experience of stress and ill health among pupils (Due et al, 1999; Natvig et al, 1999; Torsheim and Wold, 2001a; Östberg, 2003; Låftman Brolin and Östberg, 2006). In addition, when it comes to instrumental support (help with schoolwork), an important source of support is located outside the work environment, namely parents. Parental help with homework can be decisive for the child's school achievement, and the degree and quality of this support varies between children (Chen and Stevenson, 1989).

As noted by Karasek and Theorell (1990), individual characteristics, such as age and personality, can affect an individual's perception of his/her psychosocial work environment. Self-reported data on working conditions could produce conclusions about the work environment that are really attributable to individual characteristics. This is particularly relevant when studying such a heterogeneous group as compulsory school students, who, in many respects, are exposed to a relatively homogeneous work environment. One obvious risk here is that high ability students report a lower level of perceived demands because of their individual capacity to meet these demands. This problem is of course not exclusive to schoolchildren. In the adult working population, ability is likely to be highly correlated with job type via achieved education. Hence, highly educated jobholders are most likely to be found in the 'active' category of the model, whereas high ability students, on the other hand, may be more likely to end up in the 'low strain category'. Moreover, we would expect a lower share of pupils than adult jobholders to report a high degree of control, thus leading to a lower proportion of students featuring in the 'active' and 'low strain' categories of working conditions.

From an analytical point of view, the relatively homogeneous working conditions of pupils· offer an advantage by reducing the risk of health-related selection into the hierarchical structure of the 'labour market'. Finally, the school is a crucial setting for the overall psychological wellbeing of children and young people, and the fact that school is compulsory to the age of 16 makes it even more important to ensure that the psychosocial work environment offered by schools serves to enhance health.

Earlier studies have shown that the psychosocial work environment in school has a strong bearing on pupils' health, especially psychological and somatic symptoms. Issues that have been focused on include demand, control and support (see, for example, Natvig et al, 1999; Torsheim and Wold, 2001a, 2001b; Låftman Brolin, 2005; Gillander Gådin and Hammarström, 2003). Some previous studies have also more explicitly dealt with the combinations of these aspects. For example, a study of third and sixth graders in northern Sweden found that pupils in a 'low strain' situation had better health, measured by somatic problems, stress, tiredness and feelings of self-worth, than pupils in the 'active', 'passive' and 'strained' categories. However, the key explanatory factor for most health outcomes was relational problems with classmates (Gillander Gådin and Hammarström, 2000). A similar tendency was found in a large-scale study of 11-, 13- and 15-year-old students in Finland, Latvia, Norway and Slovakia. Thus, although control (autonomy), demands (measured as reasonable expectations) and teacher support seemed to be consistently related to students' subjective wellbeing in a multivariate analysis, emotional support from other students stood out as the single most important dimension (Samdahl, 1998). It should be noted, however, that the views and measures of demand, control and support applied in the studies carried out on this topic have varied considerably.

Outline of the study

The purpose of this study is to analyse aspects of demand, control and support in the Swedish compulsory school and their association with wellbeing among children and adolescents. Here, we will focus exclusively on the accomplishment of the *work task*. Thus, high demands mean having many assessments and tests, while high control is regarded as the opportunity to influence the schedule of this work. An equivalent restriction is put on social support; we look only at instrumental support, that is, help in accomplishing schoolwork. Emotional support from same-aged peers is thus not taken into account in our support dimension. This is because school is to a high degree a social arena. Social relations with peers are of great importance per se and the relations within this arena are strongly linked with those outside it, that is, during leisure hours (Hansell, 1985; Ray et al, 1995). In this way, emotional support in school reflects much more than the work environment. On the other hand, access to instrumental support will not be restricted to the help provided from teachers. For young children in particular, parents are an important source of instrumental support in helping with homework. The inclusion of parents will give a more accurate reflection of the child's true access to instrumental support in accomplishing his or her work. However, this inclusion is also a deviation from the demand-control-support model that inhibits our ability to interpret the results in line with this perspective. In order to be able to discern the influence of work organisation, we will first concentrate on the demand and control aspects and then, in a second step, include instrumental support. This study, one of the few on this topic, will contribute to our understanding of this area by employing a strict focus on schoolwork and by using a Swedish nationally representative sample.

Among children and youths, prolonged stress may express itself in both psychosomatic complaints and low psychological wellbeing. These are the main health indicators used in this study. However, we will also give a less comprehensive analysis that only presents results for the most extreme combinations of job characteristics for a number of health-related outcomes (all variables are described in the Appendix to this chapter).

In any analysis of health and wellbeing it is important to take gender and age into consideration. Girls generally have more psychosomatic complaints and poorer psychological wellbeing than boys (Danielson and Marklund, 2000; Haugland et al, 2001; Danielson, 2003; Due et al, 2003). Various explanations for this gender gap have been put forward, including differences in reporting, differential exposure to stressors, and certain stressors being of greater consequence for girls' health (Gore et al, 1992; Gillander Gådin, 2002; Sweeting and West, 2003).

Apart from gender differences, there are also age differences. The psychological wellbeing of older children is lower than that of younger children (Danielson and Marklund, 2000; Haugland et al, 2001; Sweeting and West, 2003). For psychosomatic complaints the age differences vary with the type of complaint.

Headaches are more common among older children, while sleeping problems are more frequent in younger ages (Danielson and Marklund, 2000). These age differences can at least in part be understood in relation to the changes occuring during adolescence, both physical, psychological and social. In this study we will conduct both gender and grade-level specific analyses.

The structural setting of the young person's family as well as the student's perceived ability in relation to classmates may act as confounders in the studied association by making the individual more or less well-equipped to handle demands (see Spivack and Marcus, 1987). Finally, although lack of emotional support and/or strained relationships vis-à-vis peers and parents are not taken into consideration in our support dimension of the demand-control-support model, this factor is known to be of importance for children's psychological health (Samdahl, 1998; Gillander Gådin and Hammarström, 2000). The influence of these three dimensions ('structural setting', 'ability' and 'lack of emotional support/strained relationships') on the studied relationship will be explored in a series of separate analyses.

Data material and methods

It is important that children and adolescents themselves are asked about their living conditions, especially those concerning self-perceived health and their situation in school. It is often difficult for parents to provide information about these matters. On the other hand, information from parents is needed to achieve a broader picture of children's welfare. Studies that include direct and extensive information from both children and parents in the same family, and for nationally representative samples, are rare. Since 2000, however, the large-scale Swedish welfare surveys of adults have been extended to include children and adolescents (see Jonsson and Östberg, 2001; www.sofi.su.se/LNU2000/english.htm).

The data used in this chapter is derived from the child supplements linked to the Survey of Living Conditions (ULF) conducted by Statistics Sweden in 2002 and 2003. These surveys consist of nationally representative samples of the adult Swedish population (aged 16-84). Personal interviews are carried out in the respondents' homes. The total response rate for each year is about 76%. Under-represented groups in the data are people born abroad, persons with low education and unemployed people (Statistics Sweden, 2003).

The child supplement consists of interviews with children and adolescents, aged 10-18, living in the adult respondent's household. Similar to the adults, they provide information about their lives in a broad sense, including conditions at school and health status. The information was gathered by an audio-questionnaire (a method earlier used by the British Household Panel Survey; see Scott et al, 1995). The total number of adult respondents with children aged 10-18 living in the household was 2,135, and the number of children 3,348. The response rate among these children was 80%. The present study will restrict itself to the 2,041 compulsory school students in grades 3-9. It was decided to exclude older students in order to avoid work environments based on ability-related allocation to secondary education. Full information on the variables used in the analyses was available for 99% of the sub-sample, leading to a final number of 2,017 respondents in this study.

This sampling procedure implies that the probability of being selected depends on the child's number of links with the adult sampling frame. For example, children with two guardians have twice the chance of being included in the sample than single-parent children. A weight that adjusts for these differences in sampling probability is therefore used in all of the statistical analyses. Another consequence of the sampling procedure is that certain children tend to be clustered together in the same household. To correct for the fact that siblings (or step-siblings) are not independent of each other with regard to background characteristics, statistical analyses are carried out using Stata's (8.0) cluster command, by means of which robust standard errors are obtained. The two main health outcome variables investigated in this study are psychosomatic complaints and psychological wellbeing. Multivariate analysis of the former is carried out by means of logistic regression, whereas the latter renders possible the use of ordinary least square (OLS) regression.

The theoretical assumptions of the demand-control-support model imply that there are several possible combinations of interaction effects, although a number of subsequent studies have failed to confirm such interactions (de Jonge et al, 2000b; Muhonen and Torkelson, 2003). Here, tests for all combinations of two- and three-way interactions between the three aspects will be carried out. Furthermore, even though there is good reason to believe that these job characteristics have a causal influence on health, it should be noted here that the data material used is cross-sectional. This means that questions about causality cannot be empirically investigated. The analyses will, however, show whether or not these job characteristics are associated with young people's wellbeing and whether any aspect, or combination of aspects, is more closely connected to wellbeing than the others. In this way the analyses will provide a basis for further investigation. For a description of the variables included in the analyses, see the Appendix to this chapter.

Results

Around a quarter of Swedish compulsory school students (27%) experience high demands in school in terms of too many assessments, tests and presentations (Table 6.1). A similar share (23%) claims that they enjoy high control, that is, that they themselves can influence the scheduling of their schoolwork. Where instrumental support from teachers and parents is concerned, as many as 85% report having this form of support from both sources. The gender differences for the three dimensions of the psychosocial work environment are very small. As may be expected, however, considerable differences are found between junior and intermediate level students (grades 3-6) and senior level students (grades 7-9).

Table 6.1: Distribution (%) of demand, control, support, psychosomatic complaints and psychological wellbeing (mean) by gender and grade (*n*=2,017)

	All	Boys	Girls	Grade 3-6	Grade 7-9
High demand	27	27	28	18	40
High control	23	23	24	12	38
High support	85	85	85	89	80
from teacher(s)	93	94	92	94	92
from parent(s)	92	91	93	95	87
Psychosomatic complaints	7	4	10	7	7
Psychological wellbeing (mean)	7.0	7.5	6.6	7.2	6.8

About twice as many 7th-9th graders experience their schoolwork as highly demanding compared with 3rd-6th graders. Perceived control is also much more common in the higher grades – more than three times that of the lower grades. In contrast, the differences between grade levels for instrumental support are quite small, although it is somewhat less common for higher grade students to receive parental help with homework.

As for the distribution of health, 7% of the respondents were classified as having a high level of psychosomatic complaints and the overall mean of student psychological wellbeing was 7.0. However, a higher proportion of female students report psychosomatic problems. They also score lower than male students on the psychological wellbeing index. There is no difference in psychosomatic complaints between the lower and the higher grades, whereas the average score for psychological wellbeing is somewhat better for the younger students.

The associations between the aspects of the work environment and the health measures are presented in Table 6.2. As expected, high demands are associated with significantly higher odds of psychosomatic complaints and a lower score on psychological wellbeing. High levels of control and support, on the other hand, demonstrate reversed associations. Thus for example, high instrumental support is associated with a 54% decrease in the odds ratio (OR) of experiencing psychosomatic problems and a 1.8 unit increase on the psychological wellbeing scale, compared to students without such support. Adjusting for the remaining variables included in the table does not greatly alter the crude estimates for either gender or the three work environment aspects, indicating that they are all independently associated with the two health outcomes. The estimate for gender confirms that female students are at a statistically significant disadvantage for both health outcomes, even when age, year of data collection and the dimensions of the psychosocial work environment are adjusted for.

If causality is presumed, these analyses show that the three work environment aspects have independent and statistically significant main effects. Tests for two- and three-way interactions between demand, control and support were also carried out and resulted in only one statistically significant interaction term (*p*=0.012). This interaction constitutes the combined excess effect of control and support on psychological wellbeing and will be further discussed in relation to Table 6.4(b).

Table 6.2: Regression estimates for psychosomatic complaints and psychological wellbeing by gender, age, demand, control and support (n=2,017)

	Psychosomatic complaints		Psychological wellbeing	
	Crude[a]	Mutually adjusted	Crude[a]	Mutually adjusted
	OR (95% CI)	OR (95% CI)	b-coefficient (95% CI)	b-coefficient (95% CI)
Age	1.03 (0.93-1.13)	0.98 (0.88-1.10)	−0.19 (−0.28-−0.10)	−0.11 (−0.21-−0.02)
Gender				
Boys	1.00	1.00	0.00	0.00
Girls	2.67 (1.82-3.92)	2.72 (1.84-4.01)	−1.02 (−1.35-−0.70)	−1.01 (−1.33-−0.71)
Demand				
Low	1.00	1.00	0.00	0.00
High	2.26 (1.55-3.30)	2.01 (1.36-2.97)	−1.49 (−1.89-−1.08)	-1.27 (−1.67-−0.87)
Control				
Low	1.00	1.00	0.00	0.00
High	0.52 (0.32-0.86)	0.61 (0.38-1.00)	1.05 (0.65-1.45)	0.81 (0.43-1.20)
Support				
Low	1.00	1.00	0.00	0.00
High	0.46 (0.30-0.70)	0.52 (0.33-0.83)	1.80 (1.24-2.36)	1.57 (1.02-2.12)

Note: [a] Estimates for demand, control and support are adjusted for gender, age and year of data collection.

With regard to the other combinations of work characteristics, no statistically significant interactions were found for either of the two outcomes. However, interaction terms included in OLS regression models (such as the one found for psychological wellbeing) test for additive effects, whereas interaction terms entered in logistic regression models test for multiplicative effects (Kåreholt, 2000). Additional tests for additive interactions with regard to psychosomatic complaints were carried out by calculating the relative excess risk due to interaction (RERI). In the absence of interaction RERI = 0 (Hosmer and Lemeshow, 1992). For the combinations of demand/support, control/support and demand/control, the respective RERI estimates were −0.22 (95% CI −3.40, 2.95), −0.15 (95% CI −4.26, 3.97) and 1.59 (95% CI −0.37, 3.55), indicating a synergy effect between demands and control although the estimate does not reach statistical significance.

Thus, the combination of certain work aspects seems, in some instances, to be of additional importance for stress-related health. To make the size of the combined effects visible, groups that differentiate between the various combinations of work conditions are distinguished. By combining 'demand' and 'control', four types of psychosocial work environment are obtained (Table 6.3(a)), and by adding support as a third dimension, eight types are constructed (Table 6.3(b)). The distribution of the pupils over the eight categories reveals that the most favourable or 'ideal' working conditions are experienced by 15% of the students. 'Strained' working conditions are experienced by 16% of the students and only 5% are exposed to the worst combination of work characteristics, the so-called 'iso-strained' situation. The most common combination is not among these, namely

Table 6.3: Odds ratios (OR) of having three types of psychosomatic complaints within a week, adjusted for gender, age and year of data collection (n = 2,017)

(a) Demand-control model

Overall: p < 0.000

	Low demands	High demands
High control	Low-strain: 17% 1.00	Active: 6% (0.51, 3.16) 1.27
Low control	Passive: 56% (0.75, 2.48) 1.36	Strained: 21% (1.75, 5.93) 3.22

(b) Demand-control-support model

Overall: p < 0.000

	High social support		Low social support	
	Low demands	High demands	Low demands	High demands
High control	Ideal: 15% 1.00	Active: 5% (0.34, 3.30) 1.06	Low-strain: 2% (0.73, 11.12) 2.86	Iso-active: 1% (1.07, 14.33) 3.92
Low control	Passive: 49% (0.71, 2.64) 1.37	Strained: 16% (1.80, 7.01) 3.56	Iso-passive: 7% (1.47, 7.20) 3.26	Iso-strained: 5% (2.06, 10.37) 4.62

that of low demand and low control in combination with high instrumental support (the so-called passive category comprising 49% of the pupils).

Table 6.3(a) presents the OR for psychosomatic complaints according to the four combinations of demand and control adjusted for age, year of data collection and gender. In accordance with the theoretical assumptions of the model and the results presented in Table 6.2, students with 'low strain' working conditions have the lowest odds of experiencing psychosomatic problems, whereas those exposed to the 'strained' work environment exceed all other categories, with 3.22 times the odds of reporting psychosomatic problems. The estimates for the 'active' and the 'passive' work environment fall in between the two extremes and do not much exceed that of the 'low strain' category, once again elucidating the tendency for there to be a synergy effect between demand and control. Instrumental social support is added in Table 6.3(b). Of all the eight combinations, the lowest occurrences of psychosomatic complaints are found in the 'ideal' and the 'active' categories. This contrasts with the 'iso-strained' working conditions, which demonstrate a 4.62 OR of psychosomatic problems vis-à-vis the 'ideal' category. The overall conclusion that may be drawn from Table 6.3 is that a high level of perceived control does indeed seem to protect against the negative health effects of high demands. Furthermore, students with high levels of both control and instrumental support have no elevated odds of experiencing psychosomatic complaints, regardless of whether they perceive the demands in school as high or low.

Students with 'low strain' working conditions are also the most advantaged group in terms of psychological wellbeing (Table 6.4(a)), whereas those exposed to the 'high strain' situation seem to fare worst, with an average score of 2.27 units below that of 'low strain' students. However, both the 'active' and the 'passive' work environment seem to be linked to lower levels of psychological wellbeing, perhaps the former to a higher degree than the latter. When instrumental support is introduced to the model (Table 6.4(b)), it becomes evident that this is the case only among those enjoying high support. Among those experiencing low support the situation is influenced by the interaction between control and support. Students with both low support and low control report considerably poorer psychological wellbeing than students who score low on only one of these two dimensions. To some extent, hence, high control seems to compensate for low instrumental support, and vice versa. Thus, the combination of low control and low instrumental support seems to have an extraordinarily negative effect on psychological wellbeing regardless of whether demands are high or low, although the situation seems to be even worse for those who also experience high demands. Nevertheless, the most extreme values are still found for students with 'ideal' and 'iso-strained' working conditions, with the latter group reaching an average score of 3.85 units below that of the former.

Henceforth, the presentations in this chapter will refer only to the three extreme categories of 'strained' and 'iso-strained' working conditions in relation to the 'ideal' situation. The gender and grade-level specific OR of psychosomatic

Table 6.4: OLS regression estimates of psychological wellbeing, adjusted for gender, age and year of data collection (n = 2,017)

(a) Demand-control model

Overall: p < 0.000

	Low demands	High demands
High control	Low-strain: n = 346 0.00	Active: n = 124 (−1.78, −0.43) −1.10
Low control	Passive: n = 1,121 (−1.23, −0.34) −0.79	Strained: n = 426 (−2.84, −1.71) −2.27

(b) Demand-control-support model

Overall: p < 0.000

	High social support		Low social support	
	Low demands	High demands	Low demands	High demands
High control	Ideal: n = 307 0.00	Active: n = 99 (−1.92, −0.40) −1.16	Low-strain: n = 39 (−1.84, 0.59) −0.63	Iso-active: n = 25 (−2.58, −0.34) −1.46
Low control	Passive: n = 988 (−1.04, −0.13) −0.58	Strained: n = 325 (−2.45, −1.25) −1.85	Iso-passive: n = 133 (−3.23, −1.46) −2.35	Iso-strained: n = 101 (−4.89, −2.81) −3.85

complaints are presented in Figure 6.2. The percentage figures under each bar show the share of students according to gender and grade-level in each category. We already know (see Table 6.2) that female students are 167% more likely than male students to report a high level of psychosomatic complaints. Here it can also be seen that these working conditions are more strongly linked to health among girls. Girls with 'strained' working conditions have a fourfold odds of having psychosomatic problems, while the corresponding odds for those in an 'iso-strained' situation is fivefold, compared to those in 'ideal' conditions. A similar but less pronounced tendency seems also to exist among boys. These types of working conditions are closely linked to psychosomatic complaints among 7th–9th graders but not in the group of 3rd–6th graders. It is also worth noting that the share of students in each of the three work environment categories is considerably larger in the higher grades.

For psychological wellbeing (Figure 6.3), the pattern of work type differences indicates that the support dimension is of greater importance here than for psychosomatic complaints that results in larger gaps between the 'strained' and 'iso-strained' categories. The differences are clear among both boys and girls but are of greater magnitude for girls. Whereas boys in the 'iso-strained' working environment have an average score of 2.74 units below that of boys with 'ideal' working conditions, the corresponding estimate for girls is 4.76. A similar but less pronounced tendency is also noticeable in the category 'strained' working

Figure 6.2: Gender and grade-level specific OR for psychosomatic complaints for 'ideal', 'strained' and 'iso-strained' working conditions; adjusted for age and year of data collection (% refer to the share of boys, girls, 3rd–6th and 7th–9th grades represented in each category)

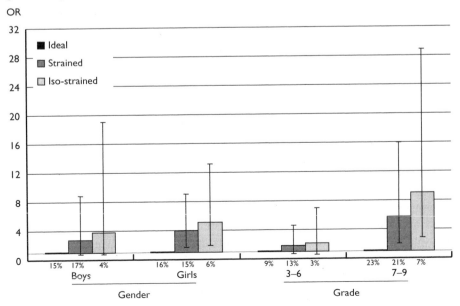

Figure 6.3: Gender and grade-level specific *b*-coefficients for psychological wellbeing for 'ideal', 'strained' and 'iso-strained' working conditions; adjusted for age and year of data collection (% refer to the share of boys, girls, 3rd–6th and 7th–9th grades represented in each category)

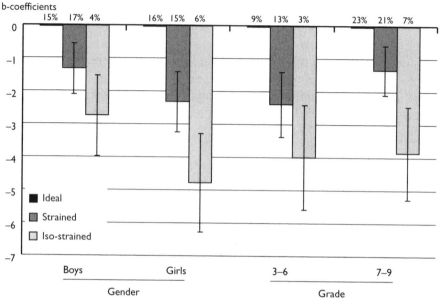

conditions. The differences between grade levels are relatively small with a clear work type patterning also in the lower grades.

Hence, the overall picture indicates that there are gender differences that put girls with 'strained' and 'iso-strained' working conditions at a disadvantage with regard to both psychosomatic complaints and psychological wellbeing. These differences also apply to boys, but to a lesser degree. Furthermore, grade-level differences, which put 7th-9th graders with 'strained' and 'iso-strained' conditions at a disadvantage, are quite strong for both psychosomatic problems and psychological wellbeing. Among 3rd-6th graders, however, no significant effect was found for psychosomatic complaints.

Table 6.5 examines whether the above-established association between working conditions and students' health can be explained or modified by (a) the structural setting of the family in which the young person is embedded, (b) self-rated ability in relation to other classmates, and (c) emotional support/strained relations vis-à-vis peers and parents (see the Appendix to this chapter). Models 1.1 and 1.2 show the corresponding estimates of psychosomatic complaints and psychological wellbeing for the 'ideal', 'strained' and 'iso-strained' situations, adjusted only for age, year of data collection and gender. Because of missing information for some of the control variables, these analyses are based on fewer numbers than those reported in Table 6.3. The baseline estimates therefore differ somewhat from the ones presented earlier. In models 2.1 and 2.2, adjusting for

Table 6.5: Regression estimates for psychosomatic complaints (OR) and psychological wellbeing (*b*-coefficient) by 'ideal', 'strained' and 'iso-strained' working conditions with stepwise adjustment for structural conditions, self-rated ability and lack of emotional support/strained relationships vis-à-vis parents and peers (*n*=1,955)

	Psychosomatic complaints (OR)				
	Model 1.1	**Model 2.1**	**Model 3.1**	**Model 4.1**	**Model 5.1**
Ideal	1.00	1.00	1.00	1.00	1.00
Strained	3.55	3.63	3.15	3.41	3.15
95% CI	(1.79-7.02)	(1.83-7.18)	(1.59-6.23)	(1.71-6.79)	(1.58-6.28)
Iso-strained	5.34	5.31	4.30	4.34	3.85
95% CI	(2.38-12.01)	(2.36-11.95)	(1.85-9.97)	(1.86-10.14)	(1.60-9.29)

	Psychological wellbeing (*b*-coefficient)				
	Model 1.2	**Model 2.2**	**Model 3.2**	**Model 4.2**	**Model 5.2**
Ideal	0.00	0.00	0.00	0.00	0.00
Strained	−1.88	−1.85	−1.50	−1.63	−1.35
95% CI	(−2.48- −1.27)	(−2.46- −1.25)	(−2.07- −0.93)	(−2.19- −1.08)	(−1.89- −0.82)
Iso-strained	−3.72	−3.61	−2.92	−2.74	−2.25
95% CI	(−4.78- −2.66)	(−4.66- −2.56)	(−3.89- −1.94)	(−3.73- −1.76)	(-3.22- −1.28)

Model 1, adjusted for gender, age and year of data collection

Model 2, adjusted for gender, age, year of data collection, social class, family type, parent's country of birth and region of residence

Model 3, adjusted for gender, age, year of data collection and self-rated ability (five-graded scale)

Model 4, adjusted for gender, age, year of data collection, lack of emotional support/strained relationships vis-à-vis parents and peers

Model 5, adjusted for gender, age, year of data collection, self-rated ability and lack of emotional support/ strained relationships vis-à-vis parents and peers

structural conditions leaves the estimates for both outcomes practically unaltered, indicating that the structural setting of the young person's family is of little importance for the association under study. When self-rated ability is introduced in models 3.1 and 3.2, however, the estimates for both psychosomatic complaints and psychological wellbeing are reduced, suggesting that part of the studied association can be attributed to variations in perceived ability. Nevertheless, the reduction is moderate and the effect of working conditions on both psychosomatic complaints and psychological wellbeing remains high and statistically significant. Thus, students with 'iso-strained' conditions are still four times more likely to experience psychosomatic problems and score 2.92 units lower on the psychological wellbeing index than students with 'ideal' working conditions, when perceived ability has been taken into consideration. Models 4.1 and 4.2 introduce lack of emotional support from friends and parents and strained relations in school and at home. For the 'iso-strained' category at least, the estimates for both outcomes are reduced, indicating that variations in support/relationships account for part of the studied association. Models 5.1 and 5.2 adjust for the combined effect of perceived ability and lack of emotional support/strained relations, both of which proved to have a modifying effect on the studied association. Although the estimates for both psychosomatic complaints and psychological wellbeing are reduced, young people in the 'iso-strained' situation have a statistically significant OR of 3.85 for psychosomatic complaints and score 2.25 units lower on the psychological wellbeing index than students with 'ideal' working conditions. A significant difference vis-à-vis the 'ideal' category also remains for the 'strained' situation.

Finally, Figure 6.4 displays a number of additional health-related outcomes for the three extreme types of psychosocial working conditions. The first one is perceived stress, something that the 'strained' and 'iso-strained' working conditions are believed to evoke. Consistent with these assumptions, 'strained' working conditions are associated with a more than doubled odds of perceived stress in comparison with the 'ideal' working situation, whereas the 'iso-strained' condition reveals a more than fourfold odds. The next two outcomes are both related to sleep. It has been suggested that sleep is an important way of recuperating from stress (Åkerstedt, 2003; Theorell, 2003), but impaired sleep can also be viewed as a consequence of prolonged stress. Students reporting that they are 'tired during the school day' and 'sleep badly' several days a week are represented fairly similarly in the 'strained' and 'iso-strained' situations. The two subsequent outcomes are based on the parent's rating of their children's psychological wellbeing in terms

Figure 6.4: Odds ratios (OR) for five health or health-related outcomes for 'ideal', 'strained' and 'iso-strained' working conditions; adjusted for gender, age and year of data collection (% refer to the overall prevalence of health-related outcomes)

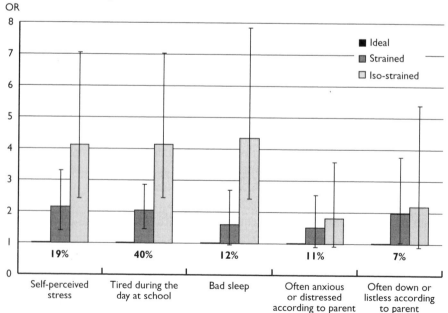

of the child 'being anxious or distressed' and 'feeling down or listless' on a weekly basis. Not surprisingly, the association between students' working conditions and their psychological health becomes less pronounced when the children's own statements about their psychological health are replaced by their parents' ratings. Nevertheless, these findings give further support to the suggestion that the psychosocial work environment is an important determinant of health among compulsory school students in Sweden.

Conclusion

It has been suggested that high levels of control and support are powerful resources for dealing with stressful situations such as working conditions characterised by high demands. This study has shown that the vast majority of Swedish compulsory school students have access to instrumental support in accomplishing their work, while control with regard to the scheduling of this task is much less common. Lack of control and support, as well as high demands, were all associated with psychosomatic complaints and low psychological wellbeing. The combinations of these working conditions also proved to be of importance. Children with strained working conditions, and especially when such conditions coincide with low instrumental support, are those who experience the worst health. These associations held when the structural setting of the family, self-rated ability and lack of emotional support and/or strained relations vis-à-vis peers and parents were controlled for. Furthermore, students experiencing these combinations also report a higher degree of self-perceived stress and tiredness during the school day and have a higher occurrence of sleep disturbances.

Where psychosomatic complaints, but not psychological wellbeing, are concerned, a high level of control seemed to act as a buffer against the negative effects of high demands. One interpretation of this finding is that psychosomatic complaints more specifically, and to a higher degree, capture stress-related processes. This should especially be the case in this study since the measure of psychosomatic complaints defines those who have several symptoms simultaneously and experience them quite frequently. Psychological wellbeing, on the other hand, is also considered to be stress-related but is probably also to a higher degree influenced by other aspects of the psychosocial environment. For example, social support provides the means for handling stressors but might also affect an individual's self-esteem and self-confidence more directly which, in turn, can influence psychological wellbeing. Where this measure was concerned, it was rather the combination of low control and low instrumental support that gave rise to additional problems. It may be the case that both support and control can boost self-confidence and self-esteem, thereby making those who lack both of these resources exceptionally vulnerable.

The harmful combinations of working conditions were more common and more closely connected with psychosomatic problems in the higher grades. However, for psychological wellbeing, the association with these unfavourable working conditions was just as strong, if not stronger, among the lower grade students. This sharp contrast between grade levels for the two outcome measures indicates that the detrimental effects of strained working conditions are reflected in a wider array of symptoms in older students. The work situation may have more serious repercussions in higher grades when, for example, the final marks are soon to be set. If severe somatic problems develop over a longer period of time in situations of chronic stress it is also possible that the grade level differences found in this study indicate that the health-related disadvantage of strained working conditions starts in the lower grades by manifesting itself as reduced psychological wellbeing. As the students grow older and a larger proportion of them find themselves in strained situations, these symptoms may develop into more severe forms of psychosomatic problems.

The three aspects of working conditions studied here do not increase our understanding of gender differences in wellbeing. The pattern for both types of health outcome was strikingly similar for boys and girls, although more pronounced among girls. It is possible that school demands are taken more seriously by girls and stem from different expectations about the behaviour of girls and boys. It has been shown that girls are more likely than boys to make high demands of themselves, and that such demands are more closely connected with psychosomatic health among girls (Låftman Brolin, 2005). The fact that girls generally gain higher marks in school can also be taken to indicate a higher degree of orientation towards school achievement among girls (NAE, 2004b).

The sampling procedure and design of the data material create some analytical limitations that need to be recognised. First, the cross-sectional character of the data means that questions about causality cannot be empirically confirmed even though there is good reason to believe that job characteristics have a causal influence on health. Second, since the sampling unit was individual pupils rather than schools, our data does not cover school- and class-level information. This inhibits the possibility of confirming the underlying assumption that our findings are largely due to work organisation. Previous studies have shown that school class context is of importance to students' health over and above the individual level (Torsheim and Wold, 2001a; Goodman et al, 2003). Third, our findings largely rely on self-reported information from children and youths, raising the issue of negative affectivity, that is, systematic negative responses due to negative states (Watson and Clark, 1984). Based on parents' ratings of their children's wellbeing, our study could, however, demonstrate a similar but much less pronounced association with students' working conditions. Still, the limitations of this study obviously restrict the scope of inference of our findings.

It is obviously important to identify conditions that contribute to the high levels of and increase in psychological health problems and psychosomatic complaints among children and adolescents. The development is believed to be due in part to an intensification of stress in children's and adolescents' day-to-day life (Danielson and Marklund, 2000; NBHW, 2001; Torsheim and Wold, 2001a). Among the adults in school, namely the teachers, a marked increase in stressful working conditions has been reported (Hemström, 2001b; SWEA and Statistics Sweden, 2001). It has also been shown that perceived school-related stress among pupils, especially teenage girls, has increased markedly since 1997 (NAE, 2001; Danielson, 2003). However, whether or not actual changes in objective working conditions have contributed to the health development is uncertain. For example, pupils' estimations of their degree of influence in school, including decisions about how they work, have remained more or less unchanged since 1997 (NAE, 2004a). Furthermore, in a study of Finnish pupils, none of the investigated school-related factors (for example, amount of schoolwork, relationship with teachers, bullying) could explain the rapid deterioration in young people's health between 1996 and 2000 (Karvonen et al, 2005). The perception of school and of school-related factors may, however, have changed. In a study of Scottish pupils, the deterioration in girls' health was ascribed in part to an increase in worries about school performance that occurred between 1987 and 1999 (West and Sweeting, 2003). In conclusion, we do not know to what degree the actual demands, control and support in school contribute to the understanding of general health developments among children and adolescents in Sweden. There is good reason, however, to believe that they are of importance per se.

In this study, pupils' control over their work situation seemed to be an effective coping resource, even though the majority of pupils report a low level of control. Considering that pupils' participation in the planning of their daily education is a goal stated in the Swedish school curriculum, the discrepancy between this goal and actual influence is noteworthy. Ways of enhancing pupils' control over their work could provide a means for schools to promote public health further in this age group.

APPENDIX TO CHAPTER SIX

Dependent variables

Psychosomatic complaints are measured by the question 'During the past six months, how often have you had the following problems?'. The specific items used here are 'headache', 'stomach ache' and 'difficulties falling asleep'. The response alternatives are: 'Every day', 'Several times a week', 'Once a week', 'Some time during the month' and 'Less often or never'. Those experiencing all three of these complaints on a weekly basis were classified as having a high level of psychosomatic complaints. This measure, hence, corresponds to the idea that stress is a general bodily reaction that can manifest itself in several types of complaint in each individual.

Psychological wellbeing is measured by a number of questions about the individual's emotional state (inspired by the self-rating scale for Swedish children aged 7–16 developed by Ouvinen-Birgerstam, 1985). The statements included here are the following: 'I often feel sad or down'; 'I'm often tense and nervous'; 'I'm often grouchy or irritated'; 'I'm almost always in a good mood'; 'I manage to do a lot'; and 'I'm mostly satisfied with myself'. The response alternatives are: 'Matches exactly', 'Matches roughly', 'Matches poorly' and 'Doesn't match at all'. The measure was constructed as a summary index where the response alternatives, when they concern negative statements, score $-2, -1, 1$ and 2 respectively. When they concern positive statements they score the exact opposite. Consequently the summary index can vary between -12 and 12. The index mean is 7.0, the skewness -1.15 and the kurtosis 1.97. When tested in a factor analysis all items fall into a single factor dimension with factor loadings varying between 0.50 and 0.72, and the scale has a reasonably high consistency (Cronbach's alpha = 0.68). However, when conducting these tests within sub-groups, positive and negative items seemed to reflect different conditions for boys in the youngest age group. In spite of this, the scale was used for the whole sample since the overall results did not differ substantially when positive and negative items were analysed separately.

Self-perceived stress is measured by the question: 'During the past six months, how often have you felt stressed?'. The response alternatives are the same as for *psychosomatic complaints*. Respondents ticking 'Every day' or 'Several times a week' were classified as often being under stress.

Tired during the school day is measured by the question: 'During the past six months, how often have you felt tired during the school day?'. The response alternatives are the same as for *psychosomatic complaints*. Respondents ticking 'Every day' or 'Several times a week' were classified as often being tired during the school day.

Bad sleep is measured by the question: 'During the past six months, how often have you slept poorly during the night?'. The response alternatives are the same as for *psychosomatic complaints*. Respondents ticking 'Every day' or 'Several times a week' were classified as sleeping poorly.

Anxious or distressed according to parent is measured by a question in the parental interview that reads: 'How often, during the last six months, has your child been anxious or distressed?'. The response alternatives are: 'At least once a week', 'At least once a month', 'Less often' and 'Not at all'. Children to respondents answering 'At least once a week' were classified as often being anxious and distressed according to the parent.

Down or listless according to parent is measured by the question: 'How often during the last six months has your child been down or listless?'. The response alternatives and categorisation are the same as for *anxious or distressed according to the parent*.

Independent variables

Demand-control-support

Since the focus of the present study is restricted to actual schoolwork, questions directly addressing the student's schoolwork have been selected as indicators of the demand, control and support dimensions.

Demands are measured by a statement reading: 'There are too many assessments, tests and presentations'. Respondents who agreed that these conditions applied to the situation in their school (by ticking a box) were categorised as having a high level of demands.

Control is measured by the question: 'Can you be involved in deciding which days you will have homework and exams on?'. The response alternatives are: 'Yes, quite a bit', 'Yes, a fair amount', 'No, not much', 'No, not at all' and 'Don't know'. Students ticking any of the three latter alternatives were classified as having a low level of control. Thus, autonomy, rather than skill discretion, is focused on.

Instrumental social support: respondents who were classified as having a high level of instrumental support from both teachers and parents were categorised as having a high level of instrumental social support. Support from teachers is measured by the question: 'Concerning your schoolwork, do you feel you get the help you need from the teachers at school?' with the response alternatives: 'Yes, always', 'Yes, often', 'No, not very often' and 'No, never'. Respondents ticking the first two alternatives were categorised as having a high level of instrumental support from teachers. Support from parents is measured by the question: 'Who usually helps you with your homework?'. The question is followed by a list of individuals that the child could be assumed to get help from. Respondents who ticked any of the boxes 'Mother', 'Father', and for children living in reconstituted families, 'Mother's live-in partner/husband' and 'Father's live-in partner/wife', were defined as having a high level of instrumental support from parents.

Structural setting of the child's family

This dimension was measured by four variables based on information reported by parents.

Social class: five categories of social class were constructed based on the occupation of the 'highest ranking' parent/step-parent in the family according to the so-called dominance scale (Erikson, 1984). The Swedish socioeconomic classification scheme (SEI) was applied (Andersson et al, 1981). The social classes distinguished are 'higher non-manual workers', 'intermediate non-manual workers', 'lower non-manual workers', 'entrepreneurs and farmers' and 'skilled workers and unskilled workers'.

Family type is a dichotomous variable taking account of whether there are one or two adults (parents and step-parents) in the household.

Parent's country of birth is a dichotomous variable taking account of whether at least one parent (or step-parent) was born in Sweden or not.

Region of residence consists of three categories: 'big city', 'town' or 'rural area'.

Self-rated ability

Self-rated ability in relation to classmates is measured by a question that reads: 'Compared to your classmates, how good do think you are in school?'. The response alternatives were: 'Among the best', 'Better than most', 'Just as good as most', 'Worse than most' and 'Among the very worst'. The variable was used as a categorical variable in the analyses.

Strained relationships and lack of emotional support vis-à-vis parents and peers

This dimension was measured by four dichotomous variables.

Strained relationship with parent(s) and/or parent's partner are measured by four questions that read: 'How do you and your [mother/father/mother's live-in partner/father's live-in partner] get on?'. The response alternatives were: 'Very well', 'Fairly well', 'OK', 'Fairly poorly' and 'Very poorly'. Respondents who ticked 'OK', 'Fairly poorly' or 'Very poorly' on at least one of the parent(s)/ parent's live-in partner were classified as having a strained relationship with an adult in the household.

Lack of emotional support from parent(s)/parent's partner is measured by the question: 'If you are concerned or worried about something, with which person or persons do you usually talk?'. This question was followed by a list of individuals that the child could be assumed to talk to. Respondents who did not tick any of the parent(s)/parent's partner were classified as lacking emotional support at home.

Lack of emotional support from peers in school was measured by the question: 'Do you have any close friend in your school class?'. The response categories were: 'No', 'Yes, one', 'Yes, two', 'Yes, three or more'. Respondents who ticked 'No' were classified as lacking emotional support from friends at school.

Being bullied in school is measured by the question: 'How often do you usually experience the following things at school?'. The four situations presented are: 'Other students accuse you of things you haven't done or things you can't help', 'No one wants to be with you', 'Other students show they don't like you somehow, for example by teasing you or whispering or joking about you' and 'One or more students hit you or hurt you in some way'. The response alternatives for each of the four situations were: 'Almost every day', 'At least once a week', 'At least once a month', 'Once in a while' and 'Never'. If the child was exposed to at least two of these situations on a weekly basis he/she was classified as being bullied.

SEVEN

Assessing the contribution of relative deprivation to income differences in health

Monica Åberg Yngwe and Olle Lundberg

Introduction

Even though it has been argued that in Scandinavian welfare research welfare includes far more than just economic resources, the latter are, of course, a central part of the concept since income and other economic resources can easily be transformed into goods and services that are regarded as important for a good life. Although average real incomes are lower in Sweden than in the UK, for example, more generous welfare state transfer programmes result in higher incomes at the lower ends of the income distribution in Sweden (Kenworthy, 2004). This also means that income inequalities are small in an international perspective, even though they have been increasing over the past decades (Fritzell, 2001). In fact, a relatively even income distribution, both in terms of wages and disposable income, can be considered an important outcome of the Nordic welfare state model (Kautto et al, 1999). As a result, poverty rates have been low and economic differences small in Sweden compared to many other developed nations. This being said, there are nevertheless clear differences in income and economic resources between individuals as well as between social groups.

The importance of economic resources for health and survival has been stressed for a long time. And although it is easy to imagine the immense effects of poverty and its consequences in terms of hunger, lack of proper housing, clothing and medical attention, poverty of that kind is no longer a common problem in developed countries. Hence, one might assume that the association between income and economic resources on the one hand, and poor health and mortality on the other hand, would be fairly weak in Sweden and many other European countries.

Yet this is in fact not the case. A number of studies have demonstrated clear differences in health between income layers. For example, Cavelaars et al (1998) compared self-reported morbidity by income level in six European countries and found higher morbidity rates in lower income groups. Their results indicate that health inequalities by income are smaller in Sweden and Finland than in

Great Britain and the Netherlands. Since previous analyses of health inequalities by educational level and occupational class did not show smaller relative differences in the more egalitarian Nordic countries, they suggest that social policies in the Nordic countries have been more effective in reducing health inequalities in relation to income than in relation to educational or class differences.

It may be argued that income mainly reflects people's socioeconomic position. However, even when socioeconomic controls such as social class, housing tenure, education and economic position have been controlled for, Ecob and Davey Smith (1999) find that income has an independent effect on a number of health outcomes. This suggests that income is more than merely a marker for the effect of other socioeconomic variables. Even though it can be argued that adjustment for other socioeconomic factors when analysing the relation between income and health could lead to over-adjustment, it is also acknowledged as a way to isolate the independent effect of income (Rahkonen et al, 2000, 2002).

But if income is important *in itself* for health, how does this work in welfare states like Sweden? One answer is that it is not income as such that is important, but rather income inequalities. This line of reasoning can be attributed to the work carried out by Wilkinson (1986, 1992). Using data for 11 OECD (Organisation for Economic Co-operation and Development) countries, Wilkinson found an inverse correlation between income inequality and life expectancy ($r=-0.81$, $p<0.0001$) when income inequality was measured by the Gini coefficient. In his earlier works he interpreted these findings as the result of large income inequalities leading to larger shares of relatively poor. Given that these people are less healthy there will be an effect on health at population level. Later on, Wilkinson's work shifted to focus more on the independent effects of income inequality, such as social cohesion, based on the argument that the quality of social relations should be better in more egalitarian societies (Wilkinson, 1996). As noted by Lynch et al (2004), more recent data on a larger number of countries have failed to replicate these earlier findings.

Today, the discussion is more concerned with attempts to distinguish between income effects on an individual level and any contextual level effects over and above the individual effect. This extensive discussion about whether, how and why income inequality is harmful to health actually dates back to the 1970s. In 1979 Rodgers presented a model of how reduced income disparities could lead to better individual health status. Income is seen as an important determinant of health at the individual level. Rodgers argued that the relation is concave, implying that health returns diminish with increasing income (Rodgers, 1979; Kawachi, 2000). In his hypothetical example seen in Figure 7.1 he includes only two individuals at different income levels – x1 being a low income level and x4 being at the top of the income distribution. The mean income of these two is x and their life expectancy is y1. Reducing the income disparities, transferring money from rich to poor, will improve x1 to x2 and reduce x4 to x3, which increases the overall life expectancy from y1 to y2. Following this example, if two countries have the same average income levels but different income

Figure 7.1: Rodgers' model of life expectancy as a function of income

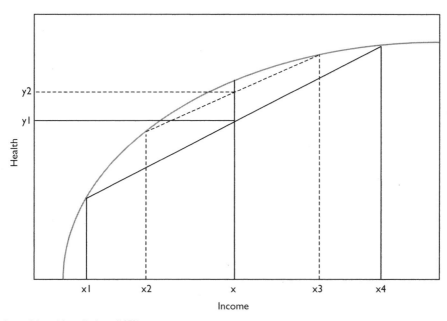

Source: Adapted from Rodgers (1979)

distributions, the country with fewer disparities would have a higher life expectancy.

Subramanian and Kawachi (2004) use the term 'concavity effect' in describing the expected relation between income inequality and average population health. They suggest that the aggregate level relation exists because of the underlying functional form of the relationship at individual level. Hence, if the relation between income and health is linear instead of curvilinear at the individual level, transferring money from rich to poor would reduce disparities in income but not lead to a better average health status in that society. Several previous studies have also demonstrated a curvilinear relationship between income and health (Ecob and Davey Smith, 1999; Fritzell et al, 2004).

If there is a substantial variation in health according to income even in an advanced welfare state like Sweden, what, then, are the reasons for it? Is it an effect of the income *as such*, in other words, is it the purchasing power that arises from a certain income that is of importance? Or, is it rather the relative position in the distribution of income that has an effect on health? In the following, we will discuss absolute and relative aspects of income, and in particular relative deprivation, as one possible factor that could explain why there are income differences in health even in Sweden.

Accounting for the association

The discussion about income and health is complicated by the fact that it mixes individual level and contextual level with absolute and relative effects of income. In many cases, relative effects have been seen as synonymous with contextual effects, and this is perhaps especially the case with relative deprivation. So how then might we distinguish between the relative and absolute aspects of income at individual level?

Absolute and relative

Before considering the effects of absolute and relative income on health, it is important to highlight problems associated with these two concepts and the ability to distinguish between them. A well-known starting point for the distinction between absolute and relative poverty is the famous exchange between Peter Townsend and Amartya Sen. In *Poverty in the United Kingdom* (1979), Townsend argues that any understanding of poverty as absolute is inappropriate, since people's needs are always conditioned by the society in which they live. Poverty is relative to the demands of society and relative to other people in society.

> Individuals, families and groups in the population who lack resources to obtain the types of diet, participating in activities and have the living conditions and amenities which are customary, or at least widely encouraged or approved, in the societies to which they belong. Their resources are so seriously below those commanded by the average individual or family that they are, in effect, excluded from ordinary living patterns, customs and activities. (Townsend, 1979, p 31)

In contrast to this, Amartya Sen (1984) suggested that poverty has an irreducible absolutist core. A now famous exchange between these two was published in the *Oxford Economic Papers* in 1985, in which Townsend argued that the 'absolute core' discussed by Sen (1984) underestimates the importance of needs other than food. Human needs are, according to Townsend, essentially social, and analyses of standards of living must take these as a starting point. In the same issue of *Oxford Economic Papers*, Sen responded to this critique by arguing:

> The characteristic feature of 'absoluteness' is neither constancy over time, nor invariance between different societies, nor concentration merely on food and nutrition. It is an approach judging a person's deprivation in absolute terms (in the case of poverty study, in terms of certain specified minimum absolute levels), rather than in purely relative terms vis-à-vis the levels enjoyed by others in society. (Sen, 1985c, p 673)

Even if we are not focusing on poverty here, it is essential to clarify the concepts of relative and absolute economic resources. Townsend's relative concept raises aspects of interest – the importance of the group or the surrounding society with which we compare our own situation. In relation to the Townsend view of demands being relative to the surrounding society, Sen (1992) later on argued that "this variability of commodity requirement shows the relativity of poverty in the space of commodities and incomes, we are still concerned here with absolute deprivation in the space of capabilities". That is, in a generally rich country it takes a higher income to buy the commodities needed to be able to take part in the life of the community. Put more bluntly, Townsend and Sen seem to agree that the human need to participate in his or her society is absolute, but that the means necessary to do that vary over time.

The debate between Townsend and Sen focused on whether poverty could be regarded as an absolute or relative concept. With regard to the relation between income and health, the interest is whether health is affected by the absolute income level or by relative income, defined as one's own income in relation to society as a whole or a particular reference group. As may be concluded from the Townsend–Sen debate, poverty in terms of reduced capabilities can be experienced on a variety of income levels, which in turn suggests that income can affect health through both absolute and relative mechanisms. In line with the last quote by Sen (1992), it is therefore reasonable to assume that one single situation or commodity could generate effects on health through both mechanisms simultaneously. For example, not being able to buy a house in a more prosperous area could generate feelings of relative deprivation that could have consequences for health. In addition, more absolute differences between areas like community safety, commuting time and food availability may also have an impact on health. Furthermore, not being able to afford food of better quality might have consequences for health both by a poorer nutritional content and by generating feelings of relative deprivation.

Neo-material/psychosocial

The difficulty in making a distinction between absolute and relative raised in the previous section is accompanied by another pair of concepts – material and psychosocial. These concepts are often discussed as two possible interpretations of the relation between income and health. Although related to the absolute and relative distinction, these two are neither contrasting nor synonymous. It might be argued that while absolute and relative are properties of income, material and psychosocial are properties of the mechanisms in the relationship between income and health.

Previous studies focusing on the separate effects of absolute versus relative income have tended to stress the descriptive distinction between absolute and relative income. While it is fairly easy to define relative and absolute income in a descriptive sense, it becomes more difficult if we want to identify the possible mechanisms generating the association. One example is Wagstaff and van Doorslaer (2000), who define the relative income hypothesis on the individual level simply as health being a function of the deviation of the individual's income from the population mean income, either defined as a national mean or the community average.

How to identify relative deprivation?

The concept of relative deprivation has been used quite extensively, although for somewhat differing purposes. Townsend (1979) uses the concept of relative deprivation in order to highlight the importance of being poor relative to the surrounding society. His definition (quoted above) could be argued to indicate social exclusion from society. Deprivation in relation to society or a group within society is important and is also discussed by others (Wilkinson, 1996; Halleröd, 1998; Stronks et al, 1998; Deaton, 2001; Eibner and Evans, 2001; West Pedersen, 2004). Some of these define relative deprivation specifically as including some process of social comparison, while others stress the effects of being poor or deprived in relation to some objective level in the group or society, not necessarily implying any comparison process. It is also possible that people adapt preferences and thereby choose reference groups that will enable them to avoid relative deprivation (Halleröd et al, 1993).

Stouffer et al (1949) originally used relative deprivation. In their studies of members of the armed forces during the Second World War they found that those with small opportunities for promotion were actually more satisfied with their promotion prospects than those with better chances of getting promoted. This seemingly contradictory finding was interpreted in terms of relative deprivation; when many around you get promoted it is dissatisfying to not get promoted. Similarly, it is easier to accept smaller opportunities when these are shared with many others.

The most influential work on relative deprivation is *Relative deprivation and social justice* by W.G. Runciman (1966). Runciman sees relative deprivation as a process in which people compare their circumstances to those of others, and he argues that this process provides "the key to the complex and fluctuating relation between inequality and grievance" (Runciman, 1966, p 6). Even though he argues that a strict definition is difficult, he defines relative deprivation as:

> A is relatively deprived of X when (i) he does not have X, (ii) he sees some other person or persons, which may include himself at some previous or expected time, as having X (whether or not this is or will be the case), (iii) he wants X, and (iv) he sees it feasible that he should have X. (Runciman, 1966, p 10)

Runciman distinguishes between three different groups that are all relevant in the process of relative deprivation – the normative group, the comparative group and the membership group. The comparative group is the group with which people compare their own situation; the normative group is a group from which the individual takes his standards and wants to be a member of. These two groups often overlap and it is in relation to the comparative group that social comparisons generate feelings of relative deprivation. The membership group (for example, working class) is the group from which the individual makes his or her claim against the comparative group (for example, middle class).

As pointed out by West Pedersen (2004), the primary goal for Runciman was not relative deprivation in the context of social evaluation as it will be discussed here, but rather as a way of understanding social and political conflict. For this reason he argued that people tend to choose reference groups fairly close to them in the social structure, while a concept of relative deprivation applicable for social evaluation must be different.

> It should be concerned also with more latent psychic, psycho-social and (possible) psycho-somatic consequences that might flow from large disparities in the command over economic resources across a population: the conscious and subconscious suffering of relatively deprived individuals, internalized feeling of failure, the potential loss of self-respect, etc. (West Pedersen, 2004, p 40)

In theory this reasoning seems plausible, but to empirically unite these dimensions in one concept seems difficult. For the purpose of using relative deprivation as a mechanism in the relation between income and health we must be able to identify which groups are important in the process of social comparison. Do we compare our income and living conditions with people at the same workplace, neighbours, friends or people living in the same city or country? Every individual is likely to have an infinite number of reference groups, but for the purpose of social comparison and social evaluation these are only important if related to feelings of relative deprivation.

Comparison process

As Deaton (2003) argues, the problem with the use of any model of relative income lies in the identification of the relevant reference groups. However, once a standard for comparison has been selected people have to (1) decide what features of their conditions to compare (income, consumption standard or some other condition), (2) perform the actual comparison, and (3) evaluate the result (Mussweiler, 2003). In order to affect health, a negative outcome of this process not only has to affect self-views but also behaviours and stress.

Here we will leave the latter parts of this process and try to elaborate a little on how a relevant comparison group might be defined empirically. Interestingly, the few studies in the field of social comparison research that directly address income or economic comparisons have assumed, explicitly or implicitly, that the relevant comparison group can be geographically defined. In other words, it comprises people in the same street, in the same neighbourhood, the same community or the same nation (see, for example, Ellaway et al, 2004; Gerdtham and Johannesson, 2004).

In principle, we would argue, there are three different approaches to defining the relevant reference group. The first, and perhaps most obvious, would be to simply ask people who they tend to compare their own conditions with. To date, however, this approach has only rarely been used. Second, we may assume that comparisons are often made with people who are similar in one way or another, in other words that the comparative group to a large extent overlaps with the membership group. This is in effect what is done when relative deprivation is calculated as the deviation from national or community averages (Gerdtham and Johannesson, 2004), or when one uses the Gini coefficient as an indicator of relative deprivation (West Pedersen, 2004). In addition to geographical proximity one can refine the membership groups by defining them in terms of similar age, similar education or social class, similar family situation, or the like. This is one of the approaches taken here. Third, it is possible to define the influence of the reference group(s) by the internalised consumption norms, and relative deprivation as the difference between people's actual consumption and the consumption standard they adhere to. This is the other approach taken here.

Defining membership groups

In studies into the relation between income inequality and health, the Gini index is an often-used measure (Subramanian and Kawachi, 2004; Lynch et al, 2004). Even though it does raise some problems, West Pedersen (2004) argues that the Gini index, as a measure of inequality, can be interpreted as relative deprivation. The key problem is that if we interpret the Gini index as relative deprivation, the underlying population is then assumed to be the reference group in relation to which each individual defines his or her social standing. One might, of course, question whether we really compare ourselves with *all* individuals in society when we make social comparisons, particularly those social comparisons that have relevance for our feelings of relative deprivation.

The crucial point here is whether we tend to make comparisons with similar others, meaning individuals close to us in the income distribution, or whether we make comparisons with individuals somewhat better off. There is also a need to clarify whether a larger income distribution affects the distance between or within relevant reference groups (see Deaton, 2003).

Apart from studies implicitly using the national or local population as a reference group, there have also been attempts to explicitly define reference groups (Åberg Yngwe et al, 2003). The reference groups were defined as people's membership group in terms of their social class, age and living region. People with an income below 70% of the mean income in the reference/membership group were considered relatively deprived. We were thereby able to study whether people with low incomes in relation to similar others (same class, age and living region) had poorer health than people not relatively deprived according to this definition. The results demonstrated an effect of relative deprivation on health, but mainly among men. When analysing the lowest 40% of the income distribution separately the relationship disappeared. The findings therefore indicate relative deprivation to be of less importance for individuals on an absolute low-income level.

We will now develop this approach. Assuming that social comparisons are the driving force behind relative deprivation, it is important to define reference groups along lines that are socially recognised and meaningful for people. The extent to which people actually tend to compare themselves with others of the same age, same social class and same living region is therefore crucial. It can be argued, for example, that the class position held, defined on basis of occupation, is not necessarily a basis for social identification any more. In order to address this issue we will here employ a measure of social class affinity as one of the dimensions creating the reference groups.

It could also be argued that position in the life cycle, rather than chronological age, is what makes people identify with each other. Several periods in life could be identified as important, but having pre-school or school-age children in the household might be more determining of consumption patterns and social comparisons than many other stages. Hence, having children under the age of 18 in the household is also a factor that defines the reference groups. Finally, we also use living in metropolitan areas as a factor defining these groups.

Consumption/deprivation in relation to norms

Even if we use here reference groups that are in part based on people's own reports of their social strata affiliation, we still do not know whether people actually do compare themselves with others who are similar in terms of social class affinity, having children at home and living in city areas. In the absence of data on who people actually compare themselves with, one might approach the problem from a slightly different angle by analysing the consumption standards people report. These standards, that is, the goods and services people say they find necessary, could be argued to reflect the norms held in their reference group. Here we can draw on the work of Mack and Lansley (1985), who introduced the method of measuring consensual deprivation.

In their concept of poverty, the 'necessities of life' are not set by a group of experts, but are rather an enforced lack of socially perceived necessities (Mack and Lansley, 1985). The method aims to relate consumption preferences to actual consumption behaviour. It does so by firstly asking respondents their views about the goods and services that one should be able to afford. In a second step, actual consumption is related to these preferences in the population. In the first step, a number of consumption items are listed and the respondents are asked to rate each item as either (1) necessary, something everyone should be able to afford, (2) desirable, or (3) not at all necessary. In the second step the respondents are asked which of these goods and services they actually do consume, and if they do not whether it is because they do not want to or whether it is because they cannot afford it (Nolan and Whelan, 1996; Halleröd, 1998).

The purpose of this chapter is not to analyse these consensual aspects. Instead of relating each item to the preferences of the population, each item will be related only to the individual's own judgement of what is necessary and what is not. Since these judgements are not made in a social vacuum, we would argue that they reflect the norms prevailing in the groups the respondent is likely to compare him or herself with. A consumption item deemed necessary is thereby socially important, and not being able to afford an item of that kind is likely to reflect relative deprivation. Therefore, if in the first step the respondent has rated an item as necessary and then in the second step answered that he or she 'does not have and cannot afford' this item, this specific item will be counted. We then compute the sum of the number of items that are necessary yet unaffordable into an index of self-rated deprivation (SRD), which we believe will measure relative deprivation. Although we do not know what the actual reference groups and norms for the individual are, it can be claimed that what is important for the individual is internalised and reflected through his or her subjective definition of deprivation.

Data and variable construction

In the first empirical part, where we analyse relative deprivation in relation to membership or reference groups, we employ data from the Level-of-Living Survey 2000 (LNU) (see Chapter One). The membership/reference groups are defined by social class affinity, whether one has children under the age of 18 in the household, and whether one lives in Stockholm, Göteborg or Malmö. This measure of social class affinity is based on the question 'People sometimes refer to the different social groups or classes in society, for example, working class, middle class and upper middle class. Do you feel any affinity to (a) the working class, (b) the middle class, (c) the upper middle class?'. There were six response alternatives for each of these three classes, namely 'Very great affinity', 'Quite a lot of affinity', 'Not much affinity', 'No affinity at all', 'Don't feel that social classes exist', and 'Don't know'.

This question generates a maximum of 18 different groups, and we therefore have to collapse categories into a more manageable number of affinity groups. The response structure contains four fairly distinct categories, namely those with very great or quite a lot of affinity to (1) the working class, (2) the working class *and* the middle class, (3) the middle class *and* the upper middle class (including those with affinity to only one of those), and (4) all of the classes. These categories respectively comprise 16%, 30%, 18% and 12% of the population aged 25-74. In addition, there is a substantial group (24%) who do not express an affinity with any class, or who believe there are no social classes.

Unlike the other groups, it is questionable whether no or only a weak affinity to a social class can really constitute a group that is recognised and used as a reference category by its members. However, these people nevertheless have a certain common way of viewing society, and due to the size of this category it is not really an option to exclude them from the analyses. We therefore have five different groups defined on the basis of their affinity to three social classes as our point of departure for defining reference groups.

In combination with having children under the age of 18 in the household and living in metropolitan areas (greater Stockholm, Göteborg or Malmö) there are 20 categories that people are likely to identify and use as reference groups. People are considered relatively deprived if they have a disposable equivalent household income of less than 70% of the median within their own reference group.

In the part of the chapter where we analyse relative deprivation defined on the basis of consumption in relation to norms we employ data from the Survey of Living Conditions (ULF), carried out by Statistics Sweden annually. Questions about consensual deprivation were included in 1998. We have included men and women aged 25-74, a total sample of 4,442 individuals (2,191 men and 2,251 women). The non-response rate was 23.3%.

The survey listed 37 consumption items and activities for the purpose of capturing consensual deprivation. In a first step the respondents were asked whether each item is:

- necessary, something that all adults should be able to afford
- desirable but not necessary
- unnecessary
- (don't know).

In a second step, the respondents were asked, for each of the same items/activities, whether he or she:

- has it
- does not have it and does not want it
- does not have it and cannot afford
- it is not a relevant question
- (don't know).

Examples of items are 'Save at least SEK500 a month', 'Private pension insurance', 'A holiday away from home for one week a year, not with relatives or friends', 'Dental care once a year', and 'Friends and family for a meal once a month'. When computing the SRD index, we count all the items that the individual has said are necessary and something that all adults should be able to afford but cannot personally afford.

Several variables are introduced in the analyses in order to adjust for confounding or to test mediating factors. Gender is a key factor, although the discussion around income and health to date has generally ignored potential gender differences. We perform all analyses separately for men and women. We also control for age and social class in order to adjust for important possible confounding.

Income is a key factor for our analyses, both as a part of the definition of relative deprivation in relation to an individual's membership group, as well as in the attempt to clarify the role of relative deprivation per se. The income measure used is equivalent disposable income, calculated on the basis of household income after taxes and transfers. In order to make the disposable household income comparable between households of different size and composition, an equivalence scale is used that gives the first adult a weight of 1, the second adult a weight of 0.55 and children a weight of 0.47. In the analysis of SRD defined on basis of consumption in relation to norms, we instead controlled for access to a cash margin. This is based on a question about the ability to raise a larger sum of money (SEK13,000) within a week.

Two measures of poor health are used, namely less than good self-rated health (SRH) and a question about anxiety. SRH is a widely used general measure of health, while the anxiety measure is less well known. It is used here because it is the only item from the index of psychological distress (see Chapter Two) that is also included in the ULF data. While it is based on a single question ('Do you possibly have any of these: inconvenience with nervousness, uneasiness and anxiety?') with three response alternatives ('Yes, severe problems', 'Yes, light problems', 'No'), it has been shown to have strong predictive validity (Ringbäck Weitoft and Rosén 2005).

Results

As discussed at length above, there is no indisputable way of empirically defining relative deprivation. We therefore test two different approaches. The first step is to analyse the possible effects of relative deprivation defined as low income within groups that people are likely to identify themselves with. We therefore assume that the membership group is also the reference group. In the second step, rather than defining a group, we suggest that goods and services that people themselves claim are necessary and something everyone should be able to afford reflect the standard in the group they tend to compare themselves with. Being unable to afford such goods and services should therefore constitute relative deprivation.

Deprivation relative to the membership group

In Table 7.1 we present the percentage of relatively deprived by gender, age and social class, as well as the prevalence of reporting less than good SRH and anxiety

Table 7.1: Percentage relatively deprived[a] (in relation to membership group) and prevalence of poor health among relatively deprived and non-deprived people, by gender, age group and social class (n=4,502)

	% relatively deprived	SRH less than good among:		Anxiety among:	
		Relatively deprived	Non-deprived	Relatively deprived	Non-deprived
All	20.1	37.5	24.6	21.4	10.9
Gender					
Men	17.6	35.5	22.1	17.3	7.2
Women	22.6	39.0	27.3	24.7	14.9
Age group					
25-29	29.9	19.8	12.8	18.5	7.6
30-34	23.2	27.6	13.0	24.1	12.5
35-39	23.4	28.4	16.4	16.5	13.5
40-44	18.8	35.7	22.8	22.6	15.1
45-49	13.4	35.9	20.2	23.4	10.2
50-54	12.3	37.3	27.3	19.4	9.7
55-59	9.8	45.6	33.6	32.6	10.6
60-64	13.3	58.3	38.7	31.3	10.5
65-69	26.0	59.8	37.3	18.3	10.3
70-74	38.8	58.1	38.6	21.0	7.2
Social class					
Upper non-manual	15.0	34.9	16.1	27.4	9.3
Intermediate non-manual	12.2	23.9	20.0	22.1	10.0
Lower non-manual	16.8	36.9	22.2	19.8	12.9
Skilled manual worker	21.1	40.3	26.2	21.4	7.9
Unskilled manual worker	27.8	44.6	35.0	24.5	15.0
Self-employed, farmers	31.6	33.3	23.3	10.9	9.3

Note:[a] <70% of median equivalent household income in one's reference category.

among deprived and non-deprived people in these population groups. Overall, a fifth of those aged 25-74 are relatively deprived in the sense that they have an equivalent disposable income of less than 70% of the median in their reference category. In other words, they have a low household income in relation to others who are identical to themselves in terms of class affinity, children under 18 and residence in metropolitan areas. Relative deprivation, defined this way, is most common among women, people below 40 and above 65, and among workers and self-employed people. This sociodemographic pattern does not, however, differ much from low incomes in general.

There are clear differences in less than good SRH and anxiety between genders and age groups, as well as very clear differences between deprived and non-deprived people within these groups. Without exception, more of the deprived report poor health, and in many instances the difference between deprived and non-deprived people is very large.

As indicated above, however, it is far from evident that the differences in health reported here are the results of unfavourable outcomes of social comparisons.

A major reason for this is that there is a strong relationship between household income and relative deprivation defined in this way (Table 7.2). The mean equivalent disposable household income among deprived people is just below SEK80,000, while the mean among non-deprived people is above SEK184,000.

Thus, there is a great difference in purchasing power between these two groups, and this brings the issue of absolute and relative income to the forefront. Is it money *as such* and the goods and services that it can buy that is important for health, or is it the *relative* value of this money that affects health through social comparisons of status or fair rewards? Or rather, what is the relative importance of the material and immaterial aspects of income? In an attempt to address these issues, we analyse the odds of being ill among the relatively deprived in relation to non-deprived people, both with and without control for income.

In model 1 we present the sex-specific OR (odds ratios) of being ill with control for age only. Being relatively deprived is associated with an increased odds of having less than good SRH of 2.28 among men as compared to non-deprived men, while the corresponding OR among women is 1.76. For both men and women relative deprivation is clearly related to poorer health, but the relationship is clearly stronger among men. This also holds true for anxiety.

Table 7.2: Equivalent disposable income (SEK) among relatively deprived[a] and non-deprived people: men and women aged 25-74 (2000)

	Men		Women	
	Relatively deprived	**Non-deprived**	**Relatively deprived**	**Non-deprived**
Mean	78,728	184,563	79,954	184,461
SD	26,974	113,412	25,753	118,412
n	394	1,841	501	1,716

Note: [a] <70% of median equivalent household income in one's reference category.

Table 7.3: Odds ratios (OR) for SRH less than good and anxiety, for relatively deprived[a] compared to non-deprived people: men and women aged 25-74 (2000)

	Model 1	Model 2	Model 3
	OR (95% CI)	OR (95% CI)	OR (95% CI)
SRH less than good			
Men	2.28 (1.78-2.92)	1.78 (1.32-2.39)	1.84 (1.36-2.49)
Women	1.76 (1.41-2.18)	0.99 (0.75-1.31)	1.03 (0.78-1.36)
Anxiety			
Men	2.73 (1.98-3.77)	2.61 (1.63-4.18)	2.59 (1.61-4.16)
Women	1.91 (1.49-2.45)	1.24 (0.89-1.73)	1.23 (0.88-1.72)

Note: [a] <70% of median equivalent household income in one's reference category.

Model 1, adjusted for age

Model 2, adjusted for age, income and income squared

Model 3, adjusted for age, income, income squared and social class

Turning to model 2, where equivalent disposable household income as well as the quadratic term is included, we see that the association between relative deprivation and poor health is reduced among men, but also that a substantial association remains. For anxiety the reduction in the OR caused by including income in the model is actually only marginal. Among women, however, the association between relative deprivation and ill health is entirely a spurious effect caused by income as such. This is clear from the sharp reduction in OR from model 1 to model 2. In model 3 we also include social class, which does not alter the OR in any substantial way. These analyses, therefore, suggest that relative deprivation plays a role for health in addition to income among men, but not among women.

Self-rated deprivation

Table 7.4 shows the percentage of men and women reporting SRD on 1 to 5 items. Seventy-four per cent of men and 70.3% of women do not report being deprived of any of the included items. Only around 3% of men and women report being deprived of 5 or more items. In the analyses, the group that has missing value on the SRD variable will also be presented, since this group consists of around 5%. Individuals who have missing value on at least one of the 37 included items were coded as having missing value on the SRD variable.

Figures 7.2 and 7.3 present the prevalence of less than good SRH and anxiety among men and women in groups of SRD. For both health measures the prevalence increases with increasing deprivation. Among those who do not have five or more items, about 50% of women reported less than good SRH and anxiety. A gender difference was found for both health measures, with women being more likely to report both less than good SRH and anxiety.

Table 7.5(a) shows OR for less than good SRH across groups of SRD, stratified by gender. For both men and women the gradient becomes steeper when we adjust for age (model 2) compared to the unadjusted model 1. The reason for this is that younger age groups are indeed more deprived, but are also less likely to report ill health. In all models, and for both men and women, there is already an increased risk of poor health among those deprived of just one item. Among

Table 7.4: Percentage of SRD: men and women aged 25-74 (1998)

	Men	Women
No SRD	74.0	70.3
Deprived of 1 item	9.4	11.2
Deprived of 2 items	4.6	5.5
Deprived of 3-4 items	3.6	4.8
Deprived of 5 or more items	2.8	3.4
Missing value for SRD	5.6	4.8
n	2,215	2,267

Figure 7.2: Prevalence (%) of SRH less than good among men and women in groups of SRD, not age-adjusted

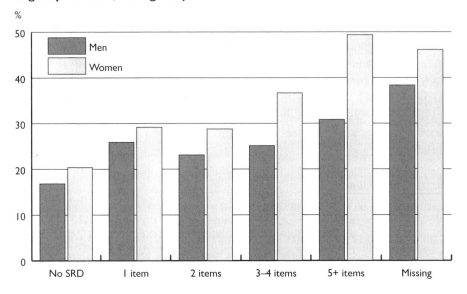

Figure 7.3: Prevalence (%) of anxiety among men and women in groups of SRD, not age-adjusted

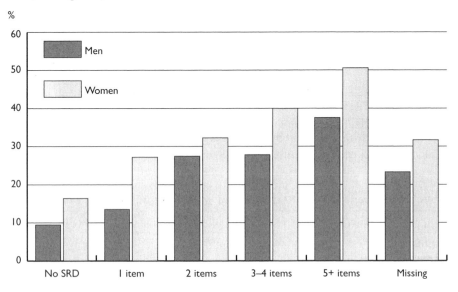

Table 7.5(a): Odds ratios (OR) for SRH less than good across groups of SRD by gender: men and women aged 25-74 (1998)

	Model 1	Model 2	Model 3	Model 4
	OR (95% CI)	OR (95% CI)	OR (95% CI)	OR (95% CI)
Men				
No SRD	1.00	1.00	1.00	1.00
1 item	1.72 (1.2-2.4)	2.01 (1.4-2.8)	1.62 (1.1-2.3)	1.78 (1.2-2.5)
2 items	1.51 (0.9-2.4)	2.11 (1.3-3.4)	1.71 (1.0-2.8)	1.56 (0.9-2.6)
3-4 items	1.67 (1.0-2.8)	2.28 (1.3-3.9)	1.75 (1.0-3.1)	1.57 (0.9-2.8)
5+ items	2.22 (1.3-3.9)	3.19 (1.8-5.7)	2.41 (1.3-4.4)	1.97 (1.0-3.7)
Missing SRD value	3.06 (2.1-4.5)	3.33 (2.2-5.0)	2.72 (1.8-4.1)	2.38 (1.5-3.8)
n	2,214	2,214	2,214	2,186
Women				
No SRD	1.00	1.00	1.00	1.00
1 item	1.61 (1.2-2.2)	2.10 (1.5-2.9)	1.92 (1.4-2.6)	1.69 (1.2-2.3)
2 items	1.58 (1.0-2.4)	2.19 (1.4-3.4)	1.96 (1.3-3.0)	1.72 (1.1-2.7)
3-4 items	2.27 (1.5-3.4)	3.02 (2.0-4.6)	2.73 (1.8-4.2)	1.77 (1.1-2.8)
5+ items	3.76 (2.4-6.0)	5.91 (3.6-9.6)	4.98 (3.0-8.1)	3.50 (2.1-5.9)
Missing SRD value	3.32 (2.2-4.9)	3.40 (2.2-5.1)	3.26 (2.1-5.0)	2.38 (1.5-3.7)
n	2,264	2,264	2,264	2,249

Model 1, groups of SRD

Model 2, model 1 + adjusted for age (10 year groups)

Model 3, model 2 + adjusted for socioeconomic groups

Model 4, model 2 + adjusted for cash margin

men there are only minor differences in illness risk as the number of items increases, while there is more of a gradient for women. As a consequence there is a greater effect of SRD among women than among men in the most deprived group. When we adjust for lack of cash margin, which is here taken as an indicator of more absolute aspects of income, an effect of SRD is still found (model 4). It can be noted that those with a missing value for SRD have an illness risk on par with the most deprived, although this is not as marked among women.

For anxiety there is generally an even larger effect of SRD (Table 7.5(b)). Here, too, the differences persist after adjustment for socioeconomic group (model 3) and lack of cash margin (model 4). Even though the wide confidence intervals indicate that the most deprived group is rather small, adjustment for socioeconomic group results in an OR of 5.06 for men and 5.38 for women. Unlike the finding for SRH, there is a gradient in anxiety among both men and women.

In Table 7.6, the OR of less than good SRH and anxiety are analysed for the highest and lowest 40% of the income distribution. To improve statistical power, SRD is in this table collapsed into a three-level variable: being deprived of no items; 1 item; or 2 items or more. The results for SRH indicate that the effect of SRD is stronger among the highest 40% of the income distribution, especially

Table 7.5(b): Odds ratios (OR) for anxiety across groups of SRD by gender: men and women aged 25-74 (1998)

	Model 1	Model 2	Model 3	Model 4
	OR (95% CI)	OR (95% CI)	OR (95% CI)	OR (95% CI)
Men				
No SRD	1.00	1.00	1.00	1.00
1 item	1.56 (1.0-2.4)	1.54 (1.0-2.4)	1.41 (0.9-2.2)	1.36 (0.9-2.1)
2 items	3.70 (2.3-5.9)	3.72 (2.3-6.0)	3.34 (2.1-5.4)	2.79 (1.7-4.6)
3-4 items	3.72 (2.2-6.3)	3.78 (2.2-6.0)	3.44 (2.0-5.9)	2.72 (1.6-4.7)
5+ items	5.84 (3.4-10.1)	6.01 (3.5-10.4)	5.06 (2.9-9.0)	3.92 (2.1-7.1)
Missing SRD value	2.97 (1.8-4.8)	2.93 (1.8-4.8)	2.60 (1.6-4.3)	2.58 (1.6-4.2)
n	2,191	2,191	2,191	2,186
Women				
No SRD	1.00	1.00	1.00	1.00
1 item	1.91 (1.4-2.6)	2.00 (1.5-2.7)	1.97 (1.4-2.7)	1.82 (1.3-2.5)
2 items	2.41 (1.6-3.6)	2.52 (1.7-3.8)	2.47 (1.6-3.7)	2.27 (1.5-3.4)
3-4 items	3.34 (2.2-5.0)	3.50 (2.3-5.3)	3.41 (2.2-5.2)	2.77 (1.8-4.3)
5+ items	5.19 (3.3-8.3)	5.56 (3.5-8.9)	5.38 (3.3-8.7)	4.38 (2.6-7.2)
Missing SRD value	2.33 (1.5-3.7)	2.34 (1.5-3.7)	2.30 (1.4-3.6)	2.13 (1.3-3.4)
n	2,251	2,251	2,251	2,249

Model 1, groups of SRD

Model 2, model 1 + adjusted for age (10 year groups)

Model 3, model 2 + adjusted for socioeconomic groups

Model 4, model 2 + adjusted for cash margin

when age and gender are controlled for (model 2). On the other hand, those with a missing value on SRD have a higher illness risk if they are among the poorest 40%. This might indicate a difference between richer and poorer respondents in the reasons for not answering these questions. Even after adjustment for lack of cash margin there is a relationship between SRD and SRH, although the estimates are shifted downwards. There is nevertheless a clear difference between the two income groups, indicating an interaction between relative deprivation as captured by SRD and income level.

Results for anxiety are again somewhat different. Although here, too, there is a clear relationship between SRD and poor health, it is not stronger among the highest 40% of the income distribution, but rather among the poorest 40%. The reason for this is not clear, but it is important to note that relationships between income, relative deprivation and health are not necessarily the same for different health outcomes.

Table 7.6: Odds ratios (OR) for SRH less than good and anxiety across groups of SRD among the lowest 40% and the highest 40% of the income distribution: men and women aged 25-74 (1998)

	SRH less than good			Anxiety		
	Model 1	Model 2	Model 3	Model 1	Model 2	Model 3
	OR (95% CI)	OR (95% CI)	OR (95% CI)	OR (95% CI)	OR (95% CI)	OR (95% CI)
Lowest 40%						
No SRD	1.00	1.00	1.00	1.00	1.00	1.00
1 item	1.43 (1.0-1.9)	1.65 (1.2-2.3)	1.45 (1.0-2.0)	1.74 (1.2-2.4)	1.75 (1.2-2.5)	1.60 (1.1-2.3)
2 or more items	1.74 (1.3-2.2)	2.21 (1.7-2.9)	1.62 (1.2-2.2)	3.92 (3.0-5.2)	4.00 (3.0-5.3)	3.23 (2.4-4.4)
Missing SRD value	4.07 (2.7-6.0)	4.71 (3.1-7.1)	3.33 (2.1-5.3)	3.98 (2.5-6.3)	4.08 (2.6-6.5)	3.62 (2.2-5.8)
n	1,787	1,787	1,759	1,764	1,764	1,759
Highest 40%						
No SRD	1.00	1.00	1.00	1.00	1.00	1.00
1 item	2.47 (1.6-3.8)	3.54 (2.2-5.6)	2.90 (1.8-4.7)	1.84 (1.1-3.0)	1.87 (1.1-3.1)	1.52 (0.9-2.6)
2 or more items	2.04 (1.2-3.4)	3.20 (1.9-5.4)	2.15 (1.2-3.9)	2.84 (1.7-4.7)	2.90 (1.7-4.8)	2.06 (1.2-3.6)
Missing SRD value	2.39 (1.4-4.0)	2.35 (1.4-4.0)	1.64 (0.9-3.0)	1.77 (0.9-3.3)	1.80 (0.9-3.4)	1.60 (0.8-3.0)
n	1,791	1,791	1,780	1,780	1,780	1,779

Model 1, groups of SRD

Model 2, model 1 + adjusted for age (10 year groups) and sex

Model 3, model 2 + adjusted for cash margin

Conclusion

In this chapter we have tried to address the issue of the extent to which relative deprivation contributes to health differences according to income in an advanced welfare state such as Sweden. In doing so, we have also tried to relate the ongoing discussion within social epidemiology to an old debate about whether or not poverty is best measured and understood as an absolute or a relative phenomenon. This illustrates that the present discussion about how to understand the relationship between income and health that exists even in advanced welfare states is neither entirely new nor restricted to epidemiology or health outcomes.

In the current debate about income and health, it has been suggested that relative deprivation is a possible mechanism, although often defined as a mechanical relationship between individual and average income (Wagstaff and van Doorslaer, 2000; Gerdtham and Johannesson, 2004). In contrast, we would argue that relative deprivation could be better understood if it is defined more directly in relation to the comparisons that people make. Here we have suggested two approaches. In the first, relative deprivation is defined as having a low income in a group that is likely to reflect central social dimensions that people identify with and use when making social comparisons. In the other, relative deprivation is defined as the individual experience of being unable to afford what he or she regards as necessities that everyone should be able to afford. Thus, our operational definitions are intended to capture relative deprivation (1) in relation to comparison groups and (2) in relation to internalised consumption norms.

Our results suggest that relative deprivation does have an effect on health as measured by the first of these techniques, although the relationship is stronger for men. In addition, among men a substantial part of the relationship remains after we have controlled for income level, but this is not the case for women. When using the second technique we find an increase in both male and female ill health with increasing degree of relative deprivation, but here the relationship is more pronounced among women. The association with relative deprivation conceptualised in the second way can only in part be accounted for by economic resources, and appears to be stronger in the upper 40% of the income distribution than in the lower 40% when analysing a general measure of health.

We can note that these results to a large degree resemble our earlier findings, despite differences in operational definitions and/or outcome measures. In a previous study, reference/membership groups were defined on the basis of occupational class, age and living region as the definition criteria for the reference groups. Despite this, and the fact that the earlier analysis was performed on data from the 1990s, the results are almost identical (Åberg Yngwe et al, 2003). An earlier study of SRD with long-standing illness as an outcome also produced very similar results to those presented here (Åberg Yngwe et al, 2006). The finding that the effect of relative deprivation appears to be stronger in the richer part of the population is also in line with earlier results (Åberg Yngwe et al, 2005). One general conclusion is therefore that relative deprivation plays a part in generating the relationship between income and health in Sweden, but that the strongest impact on health of social comparisons is to be found in the richer half of the population, where the health effects of income are smaller in the first place. Thus there is little point in trying to establish whether it is the absolute *or* relative aspects of income that produce the income–health relationship in advanced welfare states, since it is most probably a combination of both mechanisms. However, when assessing the total impact on public health of absolute effects related to purchasing power on the one hand, and income-generated relative deprivation on the other, it is important to take the curvilinear relation between income and health into consideration. If relative deprivation is most important in income layers where health is fairly good, it may not produce as many cases of poor health as do purchasing power problems in lower income strata. Therefore, income redistribution is likely to contribute to better public health, and perhaps especially so in welfare states with encompassing welfare state models with an emphasis on income-related rather than targeted social benefits (Korpi and Palme, 1998).

However, while there is a clear relationship between relative deprivation and health among men, irrespective of how relative deprivation is measured, the results are less conclusive for women. When relative deprivation is defined in terms of a low income vis-à-vis one's membership group, health differences between deprived and non-deprived people are smaller among women than among men. Moreover, when one controls for income these differences are fully accounted for among women, but not among men. In contrast, when we analysed relative deprivation defined on the basis of consumption items we found steeper differences among women than among men.

One substantial explanation for these findings could be that men and women make different priorities that also reflect the ways in which different aspects of income are related to health for men and for women. *If* comparisons of social status are more important for men than for women, and *if* differences in social status are in fact the essence of what is captured by the membership group approach, then we would expect to find a stronger relationship with health for men. Likewise, *if* women have more responsibility for everyday consumption, and *if* the SRD measure reflects relative deprivation in relation to internalised norms of everyday consumption, then we would expect to find a stronger relationship between SRD and health among women.

On the other hand, our findings might reflect other gender differences than the degree to which people react to status or prestige, or how they react to specific economic difficulties in everyday life. For example, actual differences in daily living conditions between men and women, even within households, could possibly play a role here. Examples of these are gender differences in working hours, household work or incomes. However, although all of these are important examples of persisting gender inequalities, it is not clear how they might explain the differences in results obtained with two different methods of capturing relative deprivation. Further studies of gender, income and health are called for.

Finally, we would like to emphasise the similarities rather than the differences in results, both when we compare the two approaches to measuring relative deprivation and when we compare men and women. The main finding of this chapter, then, is that income is important for both male and female health, and that relative deprivation is likely to contribute to part of this relationship. This does not mean, however, that Swedish welfare state institutions whose aim is to reduce income inequalities have failed. Rather, it is an indication of the tenacity of the social structures and processes that generate such inequalities.

EIGHT

Social capital and health in the Swedish welfare state

Mikael Rostila

Introduction

This chapter deals with the somewhat mysterious and obscure concept of 'social capital'. It was probably the famous books *Making democracy work* (1993) and later *Bowling alone* (2000) by Robert Putnam that started a new wave of analysing this concept. However, much of the recent research in this area can be seen as new wine in old bottles (van Oorschot and Arts, 2005) – not necessarily a bad thing, it should be said. It only indicates that aspects of the phenomenon have been analysed one or another way before.

Researchers have hypothesised that social capital could have positive implications for areas such as the economy (Putnam, 1993; Fukuyama, 1995), democracy, and how well societies function (Putnam, 1993). It has also been suggested that social capital may be linked to health and health inequalities. However, the empirical results have been contradictory (Pearce and Davey Smith, 2003). This chapter explores the links between social capital, health and health inequalities in Swedish society.

Social capital has a multidimensional character. Consequently, a number of aspects of social relations – such as informal social contacts with relatives, family and friends; general trust and solidarity between citizens in society; participation in voluntary associations (Putnam, 2000), and trust in the state and its institutions (Rothstein, 2003a) – have been included in the concept in earlier studies. This chapter mainly examines two dimensions of the concept, namely informal social contacts with relatives and friends and participation in voluntary associations that are often suggested to be important preconditions in the creation of social capital (Putnam, 1993, 2000).

It is likely that the (welfare) state plays an important role in creating social capital in society and in stimulating civic activities and social relations. Some researchers, however, claim that universal welfare states crowd out and destroy central aspects of social capital (for example, Wolfe, 1989; Fukuyama, 2000; Scheepers et al, 2002), while others do not support this notion (for example,

Rothstein, 2001; Torpe, 2003). In this chapter I will therefore discuss the central role of the welfare state in maintaining and creating social capital.

The aim of the present chapter is to analyse: (1) general changes in the levels of informal and formal social contacts in Sweden during the period 1968-2000, together with changes in the levels of social trust between 1981 and 1996; (2) differentials in the distribution of informal and formal social contacts between various sub-groups in Swedish society based on gender, class, country of birth, age and type of community between 1968 and 2000; (3) associations between informal and formal social ties and health outcomes at individual level; (4) whether these associations persist after controlling for a number of individual confounders; (5) how experience of poor informal and formal social ties over long time periods affects individual health; and (6) whether differences in informal and formal social contacts can explain possible inequalities in health between social classes or between immigrants and those born in Sweden.

Theoretical foundations of social capital

Social capital is a concept with roots that go back far in sociology. For example, there are undoubtedly similarities between social capital and social cohesion and the concepts of *gemeinschaft* and *gesellschaft* proposed long ago by Tönnies (1887/ 1957). Further, Durkheim (1897/1997) linked aspects of social capital to health outcomes when he examined solidarity and social support and the relation of these factors to suicide rates in different societies.

In modern times, Putnam (1993) is one of the most influential researchers in the area of social capital. He treats social capital as a mutual resource in society and defines the concept as "features of the social organizations such as networks, norms, and trust that facilitate action and cooperation for mutual benefit" (Putnam, 1993, p 167). Putnam means that social capital is created through citizens' active participation in organisations and groups. The most important norm that is created in these networks is mutuality. In other words, people expect that if they do something for someone else they will get something back in return later. This process leads to trust between members of society; they make the assumption that other citizens are going to follow the mutual norms.

Putnam (2000) claims further that some forms of social capital are by choice or necessity inward looking and tend to reinforce exclusive identities and homogeneous groups. He calls this *bonding* social capital, and this form is good for underpinning specific reciprocity and mobilising solidarity. Other networks are outward looking and encompass people across diverse social cleavages. These *bridging* social networks are good links to external assets and enable information diffusion. Putnam also talks about *machers*[1] when he refers to those people who invest a lot of time in formal organisations, like voluntary associations, and *schmoozers* when he refers to people who spend many hours in informal conversations and communion with relatives and friends. He claims that doing one of these activities increases the likelihood of doing the other, *machers* are often *schmoozers* and vice versa. Putnam also mentions two forms of trust, namely *thick trust* that refers to trust embedded in personal relations that are strong, frequent and nested in wider networks, and *thin trust* that refers to a general trust in people with whom you are not necessarily acquainted (Putnam, 2000). Putnam's reasoning thus implies that *machers* possess high levels of *thick trust* whereas *schmoozers* hold high levels of *thin trust*.

Harpham et al (2002) suggest that social capital has a *structural* and *cognitive* component. The *structural* component of social capital is the extent and intensity of participation in associations and other forms of social activity (for example density of civic associations, measures of informal social participation). The *cognitive* component refers to people's perceptions of interpersonal trust, sharing and reciprocity. Accordingly, Rothstein (2003a) claims that social capital has both a quantitative and a qualitative dimension. The quantitative dimension has to do with the number of social contacts that an individual possesses while the qualitative dimension concerns the degree of trust that characterises these contacts.

Other researchers suggest that social capital is largely an individual resource. Bourdieu (1986) claims that social capital is "the aggregate of the actual or potential resources which are linked to possessions of durable network of more or less institutionalized relationships of mutual acquaintance and recognition – or in other words membership in a group – which provides each of its members with backing of the collectively-owned capital, a 'credential' which entitles them to credit, in various senses of the world" (Bourdieu, 1986, pp 248-9). Portes (1998) suggests that social capital has to do with "the ability to secure benefits through memberships in networks and other social structures" (Portes, 1998, p 8). Finally, Lin (2001) claims that "social capital is defined as resources embedded in one's social networks, resources that can be accessed or mobilized through ties in networks" (Lin, 2001, p 73). Consequently, what unites Bourdieu, Portes and Lin in their interpretation of the concept is that they regard social capital as emanating from individual networks.

Finally, Coleman (1988) defines social capital as "a variety of entities with two elements in common: They all consist of some aspect of social structures, and they facilitate certain action of actors – whether persons or corporate actors – within the structure. Like other forms of capital, social capital is productive, making possible the achievement of certain ends that in the absence would not be possible" (Coleman, 1988, p 98). Coleman emphasises the importance of social capital for active action and productive activity. The difference between social capital and other forms of capital is, however, that social capital does not exist within the actors, but instead in the structure of the relations between the actors. His definition is very important, because it implies a shift from the individual consequences of social capital that dominate the approach of Bourdieu and others, as well as network theories, to consequences for groups, organisations, institutions or societies.

Is it possible to draw any conclusions from these various definitions despite the fact that they differ in many aspects? And how should we understand the possible link between social capital and health? Figure 8.1 is an attempt to

Figure 8.1:A social capital–health model

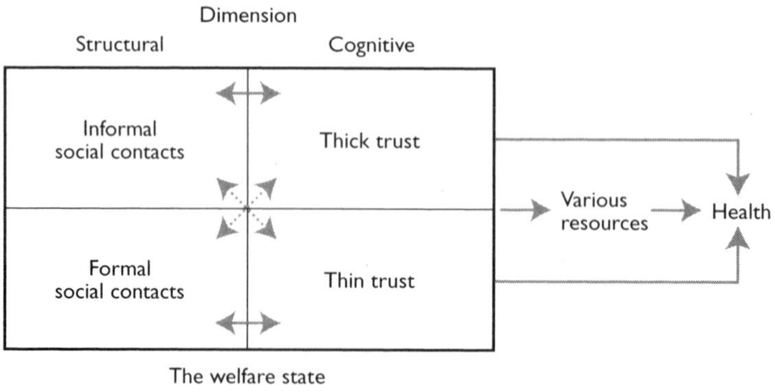

The welfare state

summarise some of the most important contributions in the field of social capital. It could also form the basis for further discussions about how different aspects and views of the concept might be related.

The model suggests that social capital has both a *structural* (quantitative) and a *cognitive* (qualitative) dimension (Harpham et al, 2002; Rothstein, 2003a). The *structural* dimension indicates that the concept has something to do with social contacts, more specifically the prevalence of different types of social relations. This might also be considered as the 'social' side of the concept. Yet the *structural* components of social capital are not social capital per se but are rather preconditions for the existence of social capital. Consequently, without social relations an individual cannot possess social capital, but can certainly possess other forms of capital like economic or human capital. This certainly makes social contacts and networks highly important ingredients in social capital, but it also links the concept with traditional network theory.

The *cognitive* dimension of the concept indicates that some form of capital, resource or benefit is derived from this social relation. This might be regarded as the 'capital' side of social capital. According to the model, the capital derived from social contacts is mainly trust. There are of course numerous other forms of benefits and resources one can obtain from social contacts that might also be regarded as capital rather than merely social trust. Nevertheless, a social relation based on trust might be considered as a foundation for the exchange of resources or benefits. If individual A trusts individual B and B trusts A, the likelihood of an exchange of resources is much higher. This reasonably holds for all types of benefit that can be obtained from social networks, such as emotional, material and economic resources. Social trust therefore makes it possible to gain access to resources embedded in social networks. Trust in itself might therefore be considered the key resource in social relations.

The model also suggests that there are two different types of precondition for social capital. Informal social contacts concern relations with, for example, friends and relatives that are strong, frequent and nested in wider networks (Putnam,

2000). These types of *bonding* relation chiefly give rise to *thick trust* (Putnam, 2000; Lin, 2001). Formal social contacts concern first and foremost social relations in *bridging* (Putnam, 2000) networks, for example voluntary associations. These networks mainly help to build *thin trust* (generalised trust) between individuals. Apparently the concepts of informal and formal social contacts are also very similar to the concepts of strong and weak ties (Granovetter, 1973). However, it is reasonable to assume that informal social contacts sometimes create *thin trust* (generalised trust) whereas formal social networks help to create *thick trust* (Lin, 2001). If, for example, people trust their family and friends they are also probably more likely to trust others in society. In line with this, some researchers suggest that good social relations with parents (informal social contacts) during childhood are important for people's level of trust in those outside family (see, for example, Uslaner, 2002). Others have found that social support from friends and relatives and neighbourhood attachment is of great importance for the creation of social trust (Li et al, 2005). However, the situation is even more complex than this. It is reasonable to assume that individuals with high levels of both thick and thin trust are more likely to socialise with other people in both informal and formal networks. This probably leads to even higher trust levels among these people. In line with this, several studies show that participation in voluntary associations leads to increased trust levels, but that there is also a selection bias, in that trust encourages people to join associations (Stolle, 2001).

The model also suggests how social contacts might be related to health and wellbeing. Individual health can be positively influenced either directly as a consequence of high levels of trust in social relations or via a variety of other health-promoting resources derived from relations characterised by mutual trust. The mechanisms linking social capital and health with the role of the welfare state will be discussed in more detail later in the chapter.

This chapter concentrates on the structural aspects of social capital and the association between these and health. In other words, the cognitive aspect is not fully discussed and the chapter focuses on the *preconditions for social capital rather than social capital per se*. However, these social contacts certainly help to create and maintain trust and other resources and indicators of social contacts can therefore be regarded as proxy measures of social capital. I therefore from now on sometimes call these contacts social capital even though they cannot be considered as social capital alone. Further, social capital is regarded as an individual resource and consequently measured at individual level. Many researchers, however, adhere to the perspective that social capital is more than the aggregated characteristics of individuals (Kawachi and Berkman, 2000), and that social capital is a feature of social structures rather than of individual actors within the social structure (Coleman, 1988; Lochner et al, 1999). Still it could be expected that individuals living in a social structure with high levels of social capital to some extent reflect that fact by their personal attitudes and behaviours. It would obviously be an advantage to be able to measure social capital as both a contextual and an individual variable. However, with the data available in this study there was no possibility to perform contextual level analyses, although Figure 8.1 could be used to elucidate the relation between social capital and health also at the contextual level.

Welfare state and social capital

According to some researchers, social capital does not exist independently of politics and the (welfare) state. People's ability to create and maintain social contacts and civic participation is, rather, strongly influenced by the institutions and politics of the state (Rothstein and Stolle, 2003). The question is then whether there are aspects of the Swedish welfare state that support and/or undermine this. Let us briefly discuss the channels through which the welfare state and its institutions may influence the two different preconditions of social capital.

Informal social contacts

There are two competing views or hypotheses about how the welfare state might influence informal social contacts. The first group of researchers (for example, Wolfe, 1989; Scheepers et al, 2002) claim that Scandinavian welfare states release people from personal obligations, such as rights and obligations towards friends, relatives, neighbourhood and so on. This is often called the 'crowding out hypothesis' (van Oorschot and Arts, 2005). By paying taxes and voting for parties that support the welfare state, the Scandinavians turn away from their direct obligations towards people in need. Boje (1996) argues that it was especially during the expansion of European welfare states in the 1960s and 1970s that civil society was gradually shut out as a result of comprehensive welfare state intervention. The welfare state institutions took over much of the obligations and support previously located in civil society and family networks. Policy makers were, however, too optimistic, and by the end of 1980s many welfare institutions and services had been privatised. This development has to some extent led to the destruction of both informal and formal social ties according to Boje. Scheepers et al (2002) examine this hypothesis empirically in a study that analyses differences in the levels of informal social contacts in different types of welfare state regimes. According to this study, universal welfare state regimes, like the social democratic ones, which are supposed to produce strong individual independence from networks such as family and friends, have the lowest levels of informal social contacts of all types of welfare state. Declining levels of informal social contacts in the period 1968-2000 might therefore be expected in Sweden, provided that the crowding out hypothesis is true.

Others claim the opposite, namely that the social democratic welfare state is the result of a society with traditionally strong norms of social trust and mutual reciprocity and that fears about the Scandinavian type of welfare state destroying moral obligations towards family, relatives and friends are unwarranted (Rothstein, 1998). This school of thought believes that well-developed welfare states create the structural and cultural conditions for a flourishing and multiform civil society.

These welfare states offer people financial resources and free time to actively develop their informal social ties; they set examples of taking responsibility for the good of others, and of behaving reliably and impartially through, for example, fair political institutions (Kuhnle and Alestalo, 2000). It has especially been suggested that well-developed social protection systems in universal welfare states could have a positive impact on social relations between family members of different generations (Kohli, 1999; Fritzell and Lennartsson, 2005). If this last hypothesis is correct we might expect the levels of informal social contact to have remained the same or even to have risen between 1968 and 2000.

Formal social contacts

There are also two competing hypotheses about how the welfare state might influence the other precondition for social capital, namely formal social contacts. Some researchers (for example, Wolfe, 1989) argue that the civil society in Scandinavia is inhibited by the development of the welfare state, which affects people's participation in organisations, groups and so on, negatively. The development of the welfare state has made voluntary organisations either unnecessary or instruments for state politics. If a civil society exists at all, it is less important here. Fukayama (2000) has a similar thesis. He is of the opinion that states can have a serious negative impact on the social capital of their populations when they start to undertake activities that are better left to the private sector or to civil society. The ability to cooperate, he argues, is based on habit and practice. If the state gets into the business of organising everything, people will become dependent on it and lose their spontaneous ability to work with one another. If these presumptions were correct we would expect there to have been declining levels of formal social contacts in Sweden between 1968 and 2000.

These views have survived, according to Torpe (2003), but are being increasingly challenged by recent research that shows that the welfare state, instead of undermining civic spirit in society and making it unnecessary, actually supports civic institutions and practice in society, both in the private and the public sphere. The relations between civic associations and the state have, since the 19th century, been characterised more by cooperation than by conflict (Klausen and Selle, 1995). In this discourse the state and the civic organisations can be seen as partners. Torpe (2003) mentions three areas in which cooperation between the state and civic organisations can arise. Firstly, the state can provide organisations with financial support. Secondly, many tasks can be transferred from the state to civic organisations. Thirdly, the state can allow organisations to participate in the political decision-making process, which gives these decisions more support. In supporting civic organisations in these three different ways, the state can relatively easily influence formal social contacts in a positive way.

Kuhnle and Alestalo (2000) also argue that there is a positive relationship between welfare state development and civil society in Scandinavia. Voluntary associations have, for example, often actively been searching for greater state involvement. As a result, on the contrary voluntary work is no less widespread in well-developed welfare states than in others. According to empirical studies in Sweden, people's trust in others, their political engagement and their participation in voluntary organisations increased rather than decreased during the time when the welfare state was developing, and levels are generally high compared to other European countries (Rothstein, 2001). Svedberg (2001) also concludes that there is no contradiction between a well-developed Swedish welfare state and informal and voluntary activities. If this hypothesis is correct, we would expect the levels of formal social contacts to have stayed the same or even increased during the period 1968 to 2000.

Social capital and health

As mentioned earlier, the empirical evidence about the link between social capital and health has been contradictory (Pearce and Davey Smith, 2003). The results seem largely to depend on how social capital is theoretically defined and empirically operationalised. Which are, therefore, the possible mechanisms that link informal and formal social contacts with health? And which are the most important empirical studies in this area of research?

Mechanisms

The two structural forms of social capital, informal and formal social contacts, probably affect health in quite similar ways and mainly through a variety of psychological mechanisms. These networks probably affect people's cognitive and emotional states such as self-esteem, social competence, self-efficiency and self-confidence that, in turn, affect mental and physical health (Berkman and Glass, 2000).

Social contacts may also affect an individual's coping abilities and his/her experienced stress, since it can be assumed that a person with a large social network characterised by support will be less likely to experience certain types of event or situation as stressful. A person with social support will be better able to cope successfully with an event or situation perceived as stressful (Cohen and Syme, 1985; Antonovsky, 1987a). Accordingly, and as mentioned in previous chapters of this volume, the well-known demand–control model in research dealing with work and stress includes a third dimension, namely social support (Karasek and Theorell, 1990).

Social ties can also affect health by promoting social participation and social engagement. Through contact with family and friends and through participation in voluntary activities, life acquires a sense of coherence (see also Chapter Five), meaningfulness and interdependence. Social engagement may activate physiological systems that operate directly to enhance health as well as indirectly by contributing to a sense of coherence and identity that allows for a high level of wellbeing. Further, they claim that shared norms concerning health behaviours (for example, alcohol and cigarette consumption, healthcare utilisation, treatment adherence and dietary patterns), together with the distribution of valuable health information in groups, may have direct consequences for the health of network members (Berkman and Glass, 2000).

Finally, Prestby et al (1990) outline three types of benefit that arise from groups within civil society such as voluntary organisations. These are material benefits, such as wages and information; solidarity benefits, such as socialising, status, group identification, and recognition; and purposive benefits, such as bettering the community, doing one's civic duty, and fulfilling a sense of responsibility. All these benefits can be seen as positive for health and wellbeing.

The effect on health of the mechanisms presented here are probably more pronounced when the social ties in question are characterised by mutual trust. Social relations are, for example, probably more emotionally supportive and more stress reducing if they are characterised by trust. Networks with a large supply of social trust are also most likely to be successful in spreading health information and establishing norms about health behaviours as well as providing network members with material and economic resources. It is therefore highly possible that social trust is the fundamental mechanism linking social contacts with health, both directly through psychological mechanisms and indirectly through a greater number of health-promoting resources. The familiar research about social networks could then be considered as part of the chain linking social capital and health.

Empirical evidence

It is well documented that social support, mainly through informal social ties, is of significance for health and wellbeing. Berkman and Syme's (1979) classical study of the relations between social networks and mortality over a nine-year period revealed that the mortality risk among those with insufficient social networks was twice as high as among those with good social networks. They used questions concerning marital status, social interactions with family and friends and membership of religious associations. Several other studies have also found associations between social support/social networks and health outcomes such as cardiovascular disease, mental health and self-rated health (SRH) as well as mortality (for example, House et al, 1988; Olsen, 1993; Shye et al, 1995; Litwin, 1998; Berkman and Glass, 2000; Bolin et al, 2003). Yet some researchers maintain that social networks can be coercive and constitute sources of strain as well as support (Due et al, 1999).

Other studies have been more focused on formal social networks and/or the cognitive dimensions that are supposed to arise from these. Hyppä and Mäki (2001) showed that differences in SRH between the Swedish minority and the majority of Finns in Finland can be explained by differences in social capital (measured as the number of auxiliary friends, trust and membership in religious associations). Rose (2000) found that social capital at the individual level (measured by sense of self-efficacy, trust of others, inclusion or exclusion from formal and informal networks, social support and social integration) was associated in Russia with improved self-reported physical and emotional health. Further, Veenstra (2005) found that trust in other members of the community was among the strongest predictors of health in British Columbia (Canada). Poortinga (2006) revealed that individual levels of civic participation and social trust were strongly associated with SRH in a study of 22 European countries.

Yet further studies find weak or no associations between social capital and health. For example, Veenstra (2000) analysed social capital at the individual level in Saskatchewan (Canada) and found that neither levels of trust nor civic participation were correlated with health. Some other studies measuring social capital as a contextual level variable also report weak associations between social capital and health (Subramanian et al, 2002; Kennely et al, 2003).

Inequalities in social capital and health

Should we expect to find differences in the levels of informal and formal social contacts between social classes and between immigrants and the native population? And what consequences do these differences have for possible health inequalities between these sub-groups?

Immigrants probably have a large share of their relatives and friends abroad and they could also have difficulties in gaining access to voluntary organisations, since these are influenced and led by people born in the country, which could lead to less informal and formal social contacts among the immigrants. Equally, the fact that there is segregation in Sweden, with immigrants and the native population and different social classes living in neighbourhoods with differing crime rates and living conditions, could give rise to health inequalities originating in differences in levels of social capital. High crime rates have been shown to contribute to the destruction of social capital within a society or neighbourhood (Kawachi et al, 1999b). One study, in line with these assumptions, shows that immigrants have much lower levels of trust than natives in Sweden (Rothstein, 2003b).

Lin (2000), however, argues that it is not only the frequency of social contacts that matters when it comes to inequality in social capital, but also the amount and type of resources embedded in the network. He suggests that certain disadvantaged groups in society interact almost exclusively with others in the same situation (homophily). Since these networks often have a poorer supply of resources or homogeneity of resources, they offer poorer social capital. Recent empirical results confirm these assumptions (Li et al, 2005).

Few studies have examined how differences in social capital might influence health inequalities. There are, however, a number of possible mechanisms. Many previous studies have been focused on whether and how income inequalities are related to health and health inequalities (Wilkinson, 1996; Fritzell et al, 2004; Lynch et al, 2004). It has been suggested that social capital plays an important role in this discussion. A common line of argument is that income inequalities are a major determinant of mortality and health problems; growing income inequalities reduce social capital, which in turn results in poorer health (Wilkinson, 1996; Pearce and Davey Smith, 2003). Income inequalities via the destruction of social capital may therefore explain both health inequalities between social classes, since the concept of social class to a high extent is influenced by income, as well as between immigrants and natives, since immigrants often bear a double burden with the negative effects of both minority ethnic status and low social position.

Another mechanism by which differences in social capital between groups could lead to health inequalities is that higher social classes and people born in the country tend to belong to the groups that exert control over health-related behaviours such as leisure time physical activity and smoking. Lindström et al (2000, 2001) found empirical evidence to support these two hypotheses. However, further research is needed to fully understand the mechanisms that link social capital with health inequalities.

Data

The empirical analyses are chiefly based on data from the Swedish Level-of-Living Surveys (LNU) in 1968, 1981, 1991 and 2000. For more detailed information about the LNU, see Chapter One in this volume. One of the analyses is, however, based on data from the World Value Surveys in 1981, 1990 and 1996[2].

Variables

Independent variables

Two forms of preconditions for social capital are measured in the empirical analyses. *Informal social contacts* are measured with two questions about whether the respondent visits relatives or friends in his/her spare time and two questions about whether he/she in turn is visited by relatives and friends. The response alternatives are: 'No', 'Yes, sometimes' and 'Yes, often'. To qualify as having good informal social contacts, the respondent must either visit or be visited by both relatives and friends at least 'sometimes'. *Formal social contacts* are measured with questions about membership of and participation in labour unions, political organisations and other forms of voluntary association. If an individual is a member of and participates in the activities of one of these organisations at least once a year, he or she is regarded as having good formal social contacts, otherwise as having poor formal social contacts. However, in the initial analyses (Table 8.1), membership of at least one organisation is enough to qualify as having good formal social contacts[3]. This is because of the lack of information about activity in voluntary associations in the LNU in 1968 and 1981. The development of *social trust* in Sweden is also briefly discussed in the chapter. This variable is measured by the question, 'Generally speaking, would you say that most people can be trusted or that you can't be too careful in dealing with people?'. The alternatives are 'Most people can be trusted', 'Can't be too careful' and 'Don't know'. This indicator appears to measure both thick and thin social trust.

Age was divided into six categories: 18-25, 26-35, 36-45, 46-55, 56-65 and 66-75. *Country of birth* is based on questions about where the respondent was born and the nationality of his/her parents. The categories are: 'Sweden', 'Within OECD' and 'Outside OECD'. As was mentioned in Chapter Two, this labelling refers to the 'old' OECD countries. If the individual was born in Sweden, or if both parents were Swedish citizens at birth, he/she is coded as a native. If the individual was not born in Sweden and both parents come from a Scandinavian or another western country, he/she is coded as 'Inside OECD'. If the individual was not born in Sweden and both parents come from an eastern European country or another non-western country, he/she is coded as 'Outside OECD'. *Class* has been operationalised with the Swedish socioeconomic classification (SEI). This is been divided into six different categories, namely, 'Higher non-manual', 'Intermediate non-manual', 'Lower non-manual', 'Skilled manual workers', 'Unskilled manual workers' and 'Self-employed/farmers'. *Type of community* is coded according to the Swedish classification of municipalities in 1967. Stockholm, Gothenburg and Malmö areas are coded as 'Big cities', other cities with a population of more than 30,000 and urban districts are coded as 'Towns', and the rest are coded as 'Countryside'.

Dependent variables

The health indicators included in this study are psychological distress and SRH. The basis for measures of health and wellbeing in the LNU surveys is the question, 'Have you in the last 12 months had any of the following illnesses or ailments?'. This is followed by a list of about 50 items, covering the most common illnesses and ailments. To form the indicator of *psychological distress*, an additive index was computed from the items 'General tiredness', 'Insomnia', 'Nervous trouble', 'Depression', 'Deep dejection', 'Over exertion' and 'Psychiatric illness'. The answer 'No' is given 0 points, 'Yes, mild' is given 1 point and 'Yes, severe' 3 points. If the respondent scores more than 2 points on this index or if he/she reports mild or severe psychiatric illness, the respondent is given the code 'Yes' on the psychological distress indicator. *Self-rated health* is measured with the question: 'How do you grade your general state of health? Is it good, bad or something in between?'. If the respondent answers 'bad' or 'something in between' he/she is regarded as having health problems.

Results

A primary aim was to examine whether there were any changes in the levels of informal and formal social contacts in Sweden between 1968 and 2000. A second aim was to analyse whether there are differences in the distribution of social capital between various groups in Swedish society during the same period.

Table 8.1 shows that the relative risk of poor informal social contacts decreased considerably between 1968 and 1991 and then remained relatively stable between 1991 and 2000 when compared to the reference group, the mean value of the four years. This indicates that people had more social contacts with relatives and friends during the period. The table further shows that men have a significantly higher relative risk of having poor informal social contacts. There are also significant differences between age groups when it comes to this type of social capital. The oldest age group has a much higher relative risk of poor informal social contacts than other age groups. Further, those born outside the OECD are much more likely to have poor informal social contacts than other groups. According to Table 8.1, there are also clear class differences, with skilled manual workers and unskilled manual workers having the highest relative risk of poor

Table 8.1: Odds ratios (OR) for poor informal and formal social contacts between 1968 and 2000[a] (n=21,014)

	Informal social contacts	Formal social contacts
	OR (95% CI)	OR (95% CI)
Year		
1968	1.43 (1.30-1.56)	0.50 (0.46-0.55)
1981	1.20 (1.10-1.32)	1.38 (1.28-1.48)
1991	0.75 (0.67-0.83)	1.16 (1.08-1.25)
2000	0.78 (0.70-0.87)	1.24 (1.15-1.34)
Gender		
Women	0.82 (0.78-0.87)	1.38 (1.32-1.45)
Men	1.22 (1.15-1.29)	0.72 (0.69-0.76)
Age group		
19-25	1.06 (0.93-1.20)	1.18 (1.07-1.31)
26-35	0.69 (0.60-0.78)	0.72 (0.66-0.80)
36-45	0.77 (0.68-0.87)	0.68 (0.61-0.75)
46-55	1.01 (0.90-1.14)	0.68 (0.61-0.75)
56-65	1.04 (0.92-1.18)	1.14 (1.03-1.25)
66-75	1.72 (1.52-1.93)	2.25 (2.06-2.46)
Country of birth		
Sweden	0.44 (0.40-0.49)	0.68 (0.62-0.74)
OECD countries	1.00 (0.86-1.15)	0.88 (0.77-1.01)
Outside OECD	2.26 (1.98-2.58)	1.67 (1.48-1.90)
Social class		
Higher non-manual	0.78 (0.66-0.94)	0.77 (0.67-0.88)
Intermediate non-manual	0.80 (0.68-0.93)	0.56 (0.50-0.64)
Lower non-manual	0.93 (0.80-1.08)	0.86 (0.77-0.96)
Skilled manual worker	1.17 (1.03-1.32)	1.00 (0.90-1.11)
Unskilled manual worker	1.48 (1.34-1.63)	1.26 (1.16-1.36)
Self-employed/farmers	1.01 (0.85-1.18)	2.15 (1.92-2.39)
Type of community		
Big cities	1.49 (1.38-1.61)	1.31 (1.23-1.40)
Towns	0.94 (0.87-1.01)	0.87 (0.82-0.92)
Countryside	0.72 (0.66-0.78)	0.88 (0.82-0.94)

Note: [a]The multivariate analysis is based on combined cross-sectional data for 1968, 1981, 1991 and 2000. The OR describe different groups' deviation from the mean odds (1.0).

informal social ties. Finally, those living in big cities have fewer informal social contacts than those living in small cities or on the countryside.

Table 8.1 also shows that there have been major changes in the levels of formal social contacts during the period. However, the pattern seems to be the reverse of that for informal social contacts. The relative risk of poor formal social contacts increased very much between 1968 and 1981, decreased slightly between 1981 and 1991, and increased again somewhat between 1991 and 2000. The most dramatic decline in participation in voluntary associations took place between 1968 and 1981. The table also reveals that women have a higher relative risk of poor formal social contacts than men, the reverse of the pattern for informal social ties. Furthermore, it is the youngest and the oldest in particular who have poor formal social contacts. Table 8.1 also suggests that individuals born outside the OECD have a significantly higher relative risk of poor formal social contacts than those born within the OECD, and that unskilled manual workers and self-employed/farmers have fewer formal social contacts than the non-manual groups. Finally, people living in big cities have a higher relative risk of poor formal social ties than those living in smaller towns and those living in the countryside.

Because some of the group differentials in social capital could have changed between 1968 and 2000 we performed some additional analyses of the interaction between year and informal and formal social contacts respectively (not shown in the table). The main finding of these analyses is that young people socialised increasingly with friends and relatives during the period. The youngest and oldest age group, the two manual working class groups and individuals born outside the OECD are especially the categories that participated less in voluntary associations between 1968 and 2000.

Even though the main focus in this chapter is on the preconditions of social capital, it can also be interesting to look briefly at trends for the cognitive aspect of social capital, social trust. The changes in levels of informal and formal social contacts presented here would lead us also to expect changes in levels of trust, since the two phenomena are believed, theoretically, to be related. Data from the World Value Survey (results not shown in the table) indicate that in 1981 57% felt that most people could be trusted. The results also suggest that there was a major increase in levels of social trust between 1981 and 1990 (66% felt that most people could be trusted in 1991), while levels fell again between 1990 and 1996 (57% felt that most people could be trusted in 1996)[4]. In other words, the development of trust seems to follow a similar pattern to that for formal, and to some extent informal, social contacts, presented in Table 8.1. When there is a decrease in informal and formal social ties there seems also to be a decrease in the levels of trust. Other data show that during the following later period 1996-2000, levels of trust seem to have been relatively stable (Rothstein and Kumlin, 2000).

A next aim in this chapter was to examine the associations between social capital and health after controlling for several individual confounders. Table 8.2 shows the associations between the two structural forms of social capital and psychological distress and SRH, respectively, in 2000. Model 1 suggests that

---

Table 8.2: Odds ratios (OR) for psychological distress and SRH less than good by informal and formal contacts: men and women aged 19-75 (2000) (n=5,142)

| | Psychological distress | | | SRH less than good | | |
	Model 1	Model 2	Model 3	Model 1	Model 2	Model 3
	OR (95% CI)	OR (95% CI)	OR (95% CI)	OR (95% CI)	OR (95% CI)	OR (95% CI)
Informal contacts						
Good	1.00	1.00	1.00	1.00	1.00	1.00
Poor	2.12 (1.64-2.73)	1.71 (1.30-2.26)	1.71 (1.29-2.26)	2.45 (1.92-3.11)	1.80 (1.39-2.33)	1.79 (1.38-2.33)
Formal contacts						
Good	1.00	1.00	1.00	1.00	1.00	1.00
Poor	1.42 (1.23-1.64)	1.15 (0.99-1.34)	1.14 (0.98-1.33)	1.60 (1.41-1.82)	1.32 (1.15-1.51)	1.29 (1.13-1.48)

Model 1, adjusted for age

Model 2, Model 1 + adjusted for social class, country of birth, gender and marital status

Model 3, Model 2 + adjusted for informal and formal social contacts there are significant associations between informal social contacts and both health outcomes. These associations persist after controlling for several individual confounders (models 2 and 3). Further, model 1 in Table 8.2 shows that formal social ties have a significant association with both health measures. However, only the association with SRH remains significant and relatively weak once individual confounders have been controlled for (models 2 and 3).

A fifth aim was to examine how poor social capital over long periods of time influences health. Table 8.3 shows how exposure to various combinations of informal and formal social contacts between 1991 and 2000 affected health in 2000, after controlling for age and health status in 1991. In other words, the table reveals how long-term experience of poor social capital or how improved social capital during this period affect psychological distress and SRH respectively.

Table 8.3 suggests that it is primarily those with poor informal social contacts throughout the decade (poor/poor) who seem to have a high relative risk of psychological distress and poor SRH compared with the reference group of those with good informal social contacts during the whole decade (good/good). However, only the coefficient for SRH is significant. The table also suggests that those with deteriorating informal social ties (good/poor) during the 1990s had a significantly higher relative risk of both psychological distress and poor SRH compared with the reference group.

Furthermore, Table 8.3 suggests that those with poor formal social contacts in both 1991 and 2000 (poor/poor) had a high relative risk of SRH problems than the reference group. However, for psychological distress the coefficients are non-significant.

Our final aim was to analyse the contribution of informal and formal social contacts to possible health inequalities between groups based on social class and country of birth in Swedish society. Table 8.4 shows the relative risks of psychological distress and poor SRH in these sub-groups. The table also indicates

Table 8.3: Odds ratios (OR) for psychological distress and SRH less than good in 2000 by different combinations of social capital in 1991 and 2000, adjusted for age and health status in 1991, longitudinal data (n=3,689)

	Psychological distress	SRH less than good
	OR (95% CI)	OR (95% CI)
Informal social contacts 1991/2000		
Good/good	1.00	1.00
Poor/good	1.26 (0.80-1.99)	1.41 (0.92-2.15)
Good/poor	1.59 (1.05-2.40)	2.29 (1.57-3.35)
Poor/poor	1.63 (0.87-3.07)	2.56 (1.40-4.69)
Formal social contacts 1991/2000		
Good/good	1.00	1.00
Poor/good	1.38 (1.06-1.79)	1.25 (0.97-1.60)
Good/poor	1.16 (0.90-1.49)	1.25 (0.99-1.57)
Poor/poor	1.24 (0.98-1.57)	1.60 (1.30-1.98)

Table 8.4: Odds ratios (OR) for psychological distress and SRH less than good by country of birth and social class, changes in Wald statistics when adjusted for social capital: men and women aged 19-75 (2000) (n=5,142)

	Model 1		Model 2		Model 3		Model 4	
	OR (95% CI)	Wald	OR (95% CI)	Wald/% change	OR (95% CI)	Wald/% change	OR (95% CI)	Wald/% change
Psychological distress								
Country of birth								
Sweden	1.00	43.91	1.00	31.63/−28	1.00	40.44/−8	1.00	29.06/−34
OECD countries	1.63 (1.18-2.25)		1.59 (1.15-2.20)		1.63 (1.18-2.25)		1.57 (1.14-2.18)	
Outside OECD	2.11 (1.66-2.68)		1.90 (1.49-2.44)		2.06 (1.62-2.62)		1.86 (1.45-2.38)	
Social class								
Higher non-manual	1.00	17.39	1.00	17.05/−2	1.00	15.78/−9	1.00	15.17/−13
Intermediate non-manual	1.11 (0.85-1.46)		1.11 (0.84-1.45)		1.11 (0.85-1.46)		1.10 (0.84-1.45)	
Lower non-manual	1.27 (0.96-1.69)		1.25 (0.94-1.66)		1.25 (0.94-1.67)		1.24 (0.93-1.65)	
Skilled manual workers	1.16 (0.88-1.54)		1.13 (0.85-1.50)		1.14 (0.86-1.51)		1.12 (0.84-1.48)	
Unskilled manual workers	1.55 (1.20-2.01)		1.54 (1.19-2.00)		1.52 (1.18-1.97)		1.51 (1.16-1.95)	
Self-employed, farmers	1.06 (0.75-1.49)		1.07 (0.76-1.51)		1.05 (0.75-1.48)		1.06 (0.75-1.49)	
SRH less than good								
Country of birth								
Sweden	1.00	64.64	1.00	48.30/−25	1.00	55.86/−14	1.00	41.92/−35
OECD countries	1.70 (1.26-2.29)		1.65 (1.23-2.23)		1.66 (1.23-2.23)		1.61 (1.20-2.18)	
Outside OECD	2.38 (1.90-2.99)		2.14 (1.69-2.71)		2.26 (1.79-2.84)		2.04 (1.61-2.58)	
Social class								
Higher non-manual	1.00	84.59	1.00	82.21/−3	1.00	74.41/−12	1.00	72.85/−14
Intermediate non-manual	1.19 (0.92-1.54)		1.18 (0.91-1.53)		1.18 (0.91-1.52)		1.17 (0.90-1.52)	
Lower non-manual	1.64 (1.26-2.14)		1.62 (1.24-2.11)		1.61 (1.23-2.09)		1.59 (1.22-2.08)	
Skilled manual workers	1.95 (1.51-2.51)		1.91 (1.48-2.46)		1.88 (1.46-2.43)		1.85 (1.44-2.40)	
Unskilled manual workers	2.59 (1.97-3.17)		2.47 (1.94-3.14)		2.37 (1.87-3.02)		2.36 (1.85-3.00)	
Self-employed, farmers	1.73 (1.29-2.32)		1.73 (1.29-2.33)		1.65 (1.23-2.22)		1.66 (1.23-2.22)	

Model 1, adjusted for age, gender, class, country of birth and marital status

Model 2, model 1 + adjusted for informal social contacts

Model 3, model 1 + adjusted for formal social contacts

Model 4, model 1 + adjusted for informal and formal social contacts to what extent the health differences between social classes and between immigrants and the native population in Sweden are explained by informal or formal social contacts by showing the percentage change in Wald statistics[5] when the two types of social capital are included in the model. If Wald statistics decrease with informal or formal social contacts in the model, this could indicate that social capital explains some of the health inequalities within these sub-groups.

Table 8.4 shows that immigrants have a much higher relative risk of psychological distress than individuals born in Sweden. The table shows that there is a 34% decrease in Wald statistics when the two types of social capital are included in the model. This indicates that the two types of social capital together explain some of the health inequalities between immigrants and natives. However, it is first and foremost informal social contacts that are of importance for these health differentials (decrease in Wald statistics by 28%). Table 8.4 also shows that unskilled manual workers have a higher relative risk of psychological distress than higher non-manual workers. Informal social contacts seem only to explain a small part of the health inequalities in psychological distress between social classes.

Table 8.4 indicates that immigrants have far more SRH problems than natives. The two types of social capital together explain about 35% of the differences in SRH between the groups, with informal social ties appearing to be slightly more important. Finally, inequalities in SRH between social classes are shown in the table. Manual workers, self-employed/farmers and lower non-manual workers have much poorer health than higher non-manual workers. The two types of social capital explain about 15% of the differences in SRH between social classes and it is almost exclusively formal social contacts that seem to be of importance.

Conclusion

The primary aim of this study was to analyse whether there were any general changes in the levels of informal and formal social contacts in Sweden between 1968 and 2000. These types of contacts are considered to be preconditions of social capital in this chapter. Some researchers have suggested that universal welfare states like Sweden have a negative effect on informal social contacts with friends and family (Wolfe, 1989; Boje, 1996; Scheepers et al, 2002), while others are not convinced of this (Rothstein, 1998; Kuhnle and Alestalo, 2000). The results of this study reveal that informal social contacts, measured as ties with relatives and friends, generally increased in Sweden between 1968 and 2000, especially between 1968 and 1991. The welfare state seems to have a positive effect on informal social ties, maybe because it offers citizens the leisure and the resources to actively develop such contacts (Kohli, 1999; Fritzell and Lennartsson, 2005). It is also possible that the Swedish state sets a good example by taking responsibility for the good of others and behaving reliably and impartially (Kuhnle and Alestalo, 2000; Rothstein, 2001).

When it comes to formal social contacts, some researchers claim that universal welfare states have a negative effect (Wolfe, 1989; Fukayama, 2000), while others are of the opinion that they actually promote voluntary activities (Klausen and Selle, 1995; Kuhnle and Alestalo, 2000; Torpe, 2003). The results presented in this chapter suggest that membership in voluntary organisations declined between 1968 and 2000, most especially between 1968 and 1981. This indicates that some aspects of the Swedish welfare state may have a negative impact on this type of social capital. It is possible that the expansion of the Swedish welfare state during the 1960s and 1970s (Boje, 1996) made voluntary organisations either unnecessary or instruments for state politics and that they therefore lost contact with ordinary people. However we are not able to test these hypotheses empirically and we could therefore be witnessing a general trend in all modern societies. The contradictory results for the two dimensions of social capital between 1968 and 1981 also demonstrate the importance of not lumping different aspects of social capital together but rather of analysing them separately.

Our findings suggest that the trends in the levels of informal and formal social contacts follow the same pattern as those in levels of social trust, at least between 1981 and 1996. To some extent this seems to confirm the theoretical assumption, that informal and formal social contacts constitute important preconditions for the creation of social capital.

A second aim of the chapter was to analyse whether there were inequalities in the distribution of social capital between various groups in Swedish society during the period 1968-2000. The results suggested primarily that there is an uneven distribution of informal and formal social contacts between social classes and groups based on country of birth. People born outside Sweden, especially those born outside the OECD, had much lower levels of both informal and formal social contacts than those born in the country. Manual workers, especially unskilled manual workers, also had much lower levels of informal and formal social contacts than other classes. This suggests that these disadvantaged groups in Swedish society probably have poor preconditions for acquiring trust and thus also social capital.

Another aim was to investigate whether there are associations between social capital and health at the individual level and whether these persist after controlling for several confounders. Cross-sectional data from 2000 revealed associations between both preconditions for social capital and SRH, associations that persisted after controlling for several individual confounders. The results are not surprising since earlier studies have also indicated associations between aspects of social capital and SRH at the individual level (Hyppä and Mäki, 2001; Veenstra, 2005). Informal social contacts are also linked to psychological distress. Overall, informal social contacts seemed to have a much stronger effect on health than formal social ties.

The effects of long-term exposure to poor social contacts on health during the 1990s were also examined in this study. Deteriorating informal and formal contacts and poor ties throughout the decade seemed to have the strongest effect on poor health. Perhaps these results indicate something about causality, namely that it is actually social capital that affects health and not vice versa. However, causality cannot be established definitively because of the long time period between the measurements. In general, the cross-sectional character of this study makes it difficult to be certain about whether it is social capital that affects people's health and/or vice versa. People with severe health problems could very well be isolated as a consequence of their health status. This is, however, a problem common to most studies about social capital and health (Pearce and Davey Smith, 2003).

A final aim of this study was to analyse whether social capital might explain possible health inequalities between social classes and between Swedes and immigrants. The results indicate that informal social ties seem to explain a considerable part of the health inequalities that exist between Swedes and immigrants, while formal social contacts seem to explain only some of the health inequalities that exist between social classes. From a public health perspective, these results chiefly indicate the importance of the welfare state to promote informal social contacts among immigrants through providing preconditions and positive settings for such ties to develop. This might reduce health inequalities between groups based on country of birth.

As mentioned previously, it is very difficult to define and measure social capital. If there is a risk that social capital becomes everything – and maybe therefore nothing – should we perhaps consider abandoning this concept? There are at least three reasons why we should probably continue to analyse this concept and its dimensions despite criticism of the evident theoretical and empirical weaknesses. Firstly, the confusion could be even greater if social capital were sub-divided into a number of separate parts. As several studies have shown, there are strong links between different dimensions of the concept, for example participation in voluntary associations, social trust and informal social contacts. If we start analysing these aspects separately it is easy to lose our comprehensive view of how these aspects are related. It is, important to continue developing new and existing structural and cognitive measures of social capital. Qualitative methods could then be useful in establishing the validity and reliability of these measures. Secondly, we cannot disregard the fact that a number of studies have found social capital to have a variety of positive effects on individuals, societies, areas, neighbourhoods and so on, which makes continuing our research into this phenomenon worthwhile. Thirdly, the introduction of new concepts and theories in science often gives rise to confusion and debate. Researchers defend their own territories if they feel that social capital is intruding into their area of research. As Kuhn (1970) once stated, this is how the scientific world works when there is a paradigm vicissitude. He suggested that we have to accept a period of confusion and argumentation if we want to achieve scientific progress. It may well be the case that researchers interested in social capital will have to accept such a period of criticism.

Notes

[1] Machers and schmoozers are originally Yiddish concepts.

[2] For more information about the survey see www.worldvaluessurvey.org/services/index.html

[3] However, Wollebaek and Selle (2002) claim that there does not seem to be any difference between active participation and membership of associations when it comes to the creation of trust.

[4] Despite the decline of social trust, levels of trust are still very high in Sweden compared to other European countries (Poortinga, 2005).

[5] If $df = 1$, the Wald statistic can be calculated as $(B/SE)^2$. It is used to test whether the estimated coefficient B is different from 0 in the population. For a description of Wald statistics see, for example, Clayton and Hills (1993). Wald statistics had earlier been used in analysing health inequalities between sub-groups (Hemström, 2004).

NINE

'What's marital status got to do with it?': gender inequalities in economic resources, health and functional abilities among older adults

Carin Lennartsson and Olle Lundberg

Introduction

Beside the physiological ageing process, ageing is associated with significant economic and social change. The impact of these changes varies between different groups, cohorts and generations. The group of older adults aged 65 and over (old age pensioners) comprises an age span of over 30 years, and covers substantial diversity and inequality. Within this diverse group, basic dimensions of stratification such as gender, socioeconomic status and ethnicity are still present. The effect of these different dimensions on inequality of living conditions varies over the life course. They also interact more or less at different stages of life. Recently, marital status has also been shown to be an important dimension of inequality, especially among older adults (Arber, 2004).

In this chapter we aim to investigate whether present marital relationship and variation in lifetime resources contribute to economic and health inequalities between older men and older women. We will study how economic resources, health problems and the functional consequences of health problems vary between men and women according to marital status. Further, we also analyse the extent to which differences in economic resources contribute to gender and marital status differences in health and functional ability.

A number of studies have found that gender differences in various morbidity outcomes persist into later life (Thorslund and Lundberg, 1994; Arber and Cooper, 1999; Lahelma et al, 1999). Older women report more ill health and disabilities than coetaneous men, but the results are ambiguous and tend to vary according to health outcome. Older women are also more likely than older men to have limited economic resources (Arber and Ginn, 1991).

Socioeconomic inequalities in morbidity persist into the oldest ages, both in absolute and relative terms, in many, but not all, European countries (Huisman et al, 2003), including the Nordic ones (Lundberg and Thorslund, 1996b; Dahl and Birkelund, 1997; Avlund et al, 2003). In general, retired non-manual workers and those with a high income had a better health status than retired manual workers and those with a low income. This means that although older women have some social advantages (for instance, more social relationships with friends and family) over older men, they still face disadvantages in terms of economic and health resources.

Understanding inequalities in the living conditions of older adults in the light of their prior life is essential. The present living conditions of older adults are a result of accumulative processes, whereby economic, social and health advantages or disadvantages from the past accumulate over the life course and influence inequalities in old age (Kuh et al, 2003). For instance, the economic resources, both savings and in particular income, of old adults are a reflection of their main occupation and degree of participation in working life. This is especially visible in countries, like Sweden, with a pension system that is to a great extent based on prior income. Since older women in Sweden, on average, have fewer years of paid employment, are more likely to have been in part-time employments, and have on average had lower wages than men, gender differences in economic resources extend into old age. All of this results in women living longer on lower annual pensions (Ståhlberg, 1994; Palme et al, 1997).

Also important for understanding the living conditions of older adults is present marital status. Research into marital status and health inequalities has demonstrated that differences in health and mortality are dependent on marital status. In general, middle-aged adults who are not currently married appear to have poorer health than their married contemporaries (Macintyre 1992; Fuhrer et al, 1999; Fuhrer and Stansfeld, 2002; Martikainen et al, 2005). Men and women without a spouse tend to have a higher risk of mortality than married couples. Such health inequalities according to marital status are sustained into older ages, although the results become mixed and less pronounced (Murphy et al, 1997; Grundy and Sloggett, 2003; Arber, 2004).

From the research briefly outlined above we would expect to find that older women have poorer economic and health resources than older men. This is not only because they are more likely to be living in a one-person household but also because their previous roles in the family and on the labour market might contribute to variations in later living conditions. In this chapter we will focus on economic and health resources, how these resources are linked to marital status, and in what way these differ between men and women.

Demography

Sweden has one of the highest life expectancies in the world. As in many industrialised countries, increases in life expectancy are no longer due to falling mortality rates in the younger part of the population since these are already very low. Instead, it is falling mortality in ages over 65 that adds to the overall life expectancy, and this is especially true for women (NBHW, 2005a). Because of the declining mortality rates a major demographic change has occurred in the population structure; Sweden is now the first country in the world where the age group 80+ exceeds 5% of the population (482,000). The corresponding figure for the population aged 65 years and older is 17%, amounting to a total of more than 1.5 million people. There are more men than women up to the age of 62, but due to differences in life expectancy women are in the majority at higher ages. Fifty-seven per cent of those aged 65+ are women and at the age of 80 there are nearly twice as many women as men.

Differences in family formation patterns and their consequences for everyday life are crucial for understanding differences in economic and health resources between elderly men and women. The lay issue is age differences between spouses. At the time of first marriage women are on average two years younger than their husbands. Remarriages are generally more frequent among men, and when they remarry it is generally to a younger woman. In general the age disparity has increased to 5-6 years at remarriage. However, remarriages after the age of 65 are fairly rare. As a result of these trends, 41% of women over the age of 65 are widowed, compared with 13% of men of that age. Consequently, women are more likely than men to live to be old and to face old age living alone.

Structural changes in marital status in the population are noticeable not only among younger people in Sweden but also among older adults. Since 1985 the share of married and divorced men and women after the age of 70 has increased slightly while the share of widowed and never married men has decreased (Statistics Sweden, 2004). Increasing numbers of years of marriage may however not be purely positive since this can also prolong the burden of care. Many people will become chronically ill and disabled in old age and too frail to lead an independent life. This is the stage of life sometimes called the 'fourth age' (Laslett, 1987). On average, due to chronological age, men reach the 'fourth age' first within a marriage and are thus more likely to become dependent on their wives for their day-to-day needs.

Before reaching the 'fourth age' the daily lives of older adults are typically full of activities and relationships and not particularly limited by ill health and disability. Their economic circumstances also tend to be more or less secure. Despite some indication in the 1990s of a general increase in poor health, primarily in disease and functional limitations, but not disability, among the oldest old (75+) (Freedman et al, 2004; Thorslund et al, 2004; Parker et al, 2005; Rosén and Haglund, 2005), the whole group of older adults (65+) are in much better health today than they were 20-30 years ago.

Life after retirement thus usually contains several years free from illness and disability, after which come a number of more fragile years at the end of life. When, and for how many years, these two periods occur will in many respects be a question of earlier and current resources and circumstances. The main social policies directed toward older adults are the old age pension scheme and social services in the form of old age care. Depending on previous and present resources and circumstances these welfare benefits, together with healthcare, have varying implication for the living conditions of adults in later life.

Welfare state

Welfare state institutions can be divided in two major categories: 'cash' and 'care'. Among older adults the main cash category is pensions, while the care category includes old age care and healthcare.

Pensions

The foundation of the welfare state in Sweden goes back over a hundred years; one of the first breakthroughs was the general pension, introduced in 1913. The first pension reform brought the whole population into one single scheme. New legislation for a national basic pension was passed in 1946. In 1959 an earnings-related pension programme was introduced; this programme is considered to be one of the most generous schemes in the world (Kangas and Palme, 2005).

In 1999 a new pension scheme was introduced. Separate rules for specific birth cohorts were initiated in order to facilitate the transition to the new pension scheme; these do not significantly affect present-day old age pensioners (Palme, 2003). The present provision for the birth cohorts born in 1937 or earlier consists of a supplementary pension and/or a guarantee pension. The supplementary pension is earnings related and is based on earned pension points. The guarantee pension is payable to those with a low or no supplementary pension. The main purpose of the guarantee pension is to create basic security for everyone in old age. The guarantee pension is payable to those who have lived in Sweden for at least three years. The pension is liable to tax.

In an international perspective, poverty is uncommon and economic inequalities small among older adults in Sweden, both under and above the statutory pension age (Fritzell and Ritakallio, 2004). This is true both for women and men, but since the supplementary pension is calculated on the basis of earlier income there is a substantial group of women who live on their guarantee pension only.

The retirement age in Sweden is 65 for women and men alike. This reform was introduced in 1976 when the life expectancy was 77 years for women and 72 years for men. Today the actual average age for exiting from the labour market is lower, and while some groups remain working after the age of 65, many others leave much earlier, either on an early retirement pension, long-term sick leave or because of unemployment. Applied in the new retirement system is also a flexible retirement age from the age of 61. This, together with the increasing life expectancy, means that the number of remaining years of life after leaving paid employment is rising. On average, men spend 17 years as a pensioner and women 21 years (authors' own calculations from population-based data, Statistics Sweden, 2005a).

Retiring on an old age pension used to be predominantly the preserve of men and unmarried women. However, married women's increasing employment participation has increased the total number of women leaving paid work for life as a pensioner. Leaving paid work does not necessarily mean giving up work. Older adults, and especially women, will continue to have main responsibility for unpaid household work after retirement age.

Care of older adults

Swedish old age care was almost entirely confined to institutions until the 1950s, by which time the home help services had started on a small scale. Instead of offering a place in a poor house, municipalities began to offer help and support to elderly people in their own homes (Trydegård, 2000). A combination of political will and economic growth caused this popular service to expand rapidly. Thus, by the mid-1950s an official goal of Swedish elderly care was that an old person in need of support should remain at home and be supported by public services (Szebehely, 1998). Since this time, children have had no legal responsibilities for their aged parents (Sundström and Johansson, 2004). The expansion of public old age care resulted in a new living situation for both older people, their spouses and their children. Thanks to public care, older people could stay at home and receive help and support from the municipality.

In an international perspective, Sweden still has a well-developed system of municipal old age care with an integrated system of funding, assessment and supply of both home help services and institutional care. The Scandinavian countries are similar in many ways, although more recent research has revealed a significant shift in Sweden away from universalism and equality promotion towards unpaid care and more private market-based care services, leading to a segmented welfare (Szebehely, 2005).

At present, public care for older people is a needs-tested benefit. Older adults have to apply for help and a local government official carries out an assessment of their needs. The decision as to whether the older person will receive any help at all, home help or a place in special housing is based on this assessment. During recent decades geriatric wards have been closed and more emphasis has been placed on home-based care. As a result of the rising care load among older people living at home, public old age care services, via municipalities, have given priority to those with the heaviest care needs (Palme et al, 2003; Szebehely, 2005). Hence, public resources are targeted at the most frail and dependent older adults, which has transformed the home help services into a more medical form of care. Need of a more social nature, for example, social contact, are left to family and relatives, or neglected altogether (Palme et al, 2003).

In 2004, 20% of all people aged 80 and over received public home help or home nursing, 17% lived in special housing, with service around the clock, such as nursing homes, old people's homes, or group accommodation for people with dementia (MHSA, 2005).

Care and services for older adults are largely (over 80%) financed by municipal taxes, with a smaller share coming from state grants paid to municipalities. About 4% of the costs are financed by fees or rates. Most municipalities apply a system whereby the charges for services vary in accordance with a person's income and the amount of services received. The fees for home care vary between being free of charge for the least well-off pensioners and costing the market rate for the most well-off. In 2002 an upper limit was put on user fees for public home care and institutional care, which is also subsidised. As a consequence of this, one third of old age care recipients pay no fee (NBHW, 2005b).

Pensions and welfare services thus represent two important resources for older adults. Since many of them are dependent on the shape of a society's policy, the shape and extent of the welfare system have major implications for the wellbeing of older adults.

Data

To cover the whole population over 65 years of age we combined data from the 2000 Swedish Level-of-Living Survey (LNU) with data from the 2002 Swedish Panel Study of Living Conditions of the Oldest Old (SWEOLD), consisting in total of 1,229 people. The SWEOLD sample is an extension of the LNU incorporating the oldest age groups and includes all subjects who were interviewed at least once in any of the previous LNU surveys but who were over the age of 75 in 2000 and thus above the upper age bracket (Lundberg and Thorslund, 1996a; Thorslund et al, 2004). SWEOLD is a nationally representative sample of survivors from the birth cohorts 1892-1925. The response rate for the age group 65-75 in LNU was 71.2% and for the older age groups covered by SWEOLD it is 87.9%. The SWEOLD study comprised people living both in institutions and in their own homes, and both direct and proxy interviews were used. Information from proxy interviews was included in this study in order to get a complete picture of the living conditions of older adults, independent of their state of health.

Results

Economic resources

In this section we will examine gender differences in economic resources, focusing on patterns according to marital status. Economic resources have been shown to be one of the most central welfare resources because of the clear association with other important aspects of life such as health and working conditions (Erikson and Tåhlin, 1987; Fritzell and Lundberg, 2000b).

Economic resources are central since they are often easily transformed, and this is especially true for monetary resources in terms of income and savings. Nevertheless, income and savings can have different implications and meanings. Income in one sense represents 'cash flow', and relates directly to the material conditions of everyday life that may influence health in later life. A decent income has implications for the consumption of food, purchasing of medicines and caring services, opportunities for leisure activities and recreation etc. As discussed above, the pension system is constructed in such a way that incomes in later life reflect the cumulative influence of income levels throughout the life course. Savings, on the other hand, may be less important for everyday consumption but more important for economic security. Having access to an economic buffer will increase a person's ability to cope with sudden and/or unforeseen problems, and may therefore make life in old age less stressful.

To analyse differences in economic resources among older men and women of different marital statuses we employed two indicators: *equivalent disposable income* and *cash margin*. The household's *equivalent disposable income* includes both the respondent's and the spouse's income from work (if any), capital, pensions and other cash benefits as well as the taxes paid. While married or cohabiting couples often have two incomes their costs for housing, food and other expenditures are not usually twice that of single people. An equivalence scale was therefore used to adjust the income of two-person households by a factor of 1.55. This means that a two-person household needs a disposable income that is 55% larger than a one-person household in order to have the same economic standard (Jansson, 2000). Information on income was linked from a number of official registers, mainly tax records. There are consequently very few missing values for the income variable.

Public transfers in the form of pensions and cash benefits are the main source of income for older adults. The median equivalent disposable household income for the whole group of older adults over the age of 65 years was approximately SEK113,200 in 2000 (mean SEK135,500). Pensioners generally have lower incomes than middle-aged people but higher incomes than young adults, while the income distribution tends to be narrower among those aged over 65.

There are, nevertheless, clear and systematic differences in income among those over retirement age. For example, in Figure 9.1 the median equivalent disposable income is presented for married/cohabiting couples and unmarried women and men (never married, divorced and widowed taken together). As can be seen the median income is related both to marital status, age and gender. The equivalent disposable income is clearly higher among couples than among singles. To some extent this might depend on the equivalence scale chosen. If we would assume a smaller gain from economics of scale by changing to the traditional OECD scale (giving spouses a weight of 0.7 rather than 0.55) the incomes of couples (per consumption unit) would be almost similar to that of single men. However, while the equivalence scale used is not designed specifically for the older part of the population, there is no information available suggesting that the differences in living expenses between single and two-person households differ substantially between age groups. Our conclusion, therefore, is that couples do have a better economic situation in terms of disposable incomes compared to single older adults.

Figure 9.1: Median equivalent disposable household income by age group (2000)

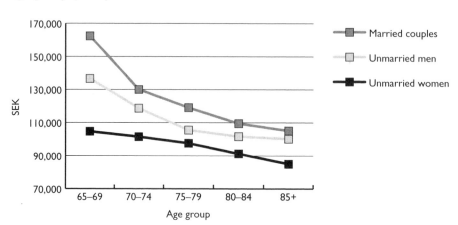

The most striking difference, however, is perhaps that between single men and single women. The difference is particularly large among the newly retired: SEK32,000 or 31%. The differences between married women and single women are even larger, and again most pronounced among the newly retired (65-69 years old).

Figure 9.1 also shows that the general income level is higher among young older adults. There are a number of reasons for this. Firstly, those who have recently retired have on average higher earnings-related supplementary pensions and thereby higher incomes than older pensioners. Secondly, many younger pensioners have insurance through collective agreements and a private insurance policy that is often paid out during the first five years after retirement. However, these explanations seem to apply to men but not that well to women – the age gradient among single women is much flatter than among single men.

Table 9.1: Distribution of marital status groups and median equivalent household income by gender and marital status (2000)

	% within each gender		Median household income SEK		
	Men	**Women**	**Men**	**Women**	*Difference men–women*
All			129,803	102,636	27,167
Marital status					
Married/cohabiting	69	38	137,925	130,840	7,085
Widow/er	16	47	116,551	95,782	20,769
Divorced	7	9	115,131	93,405	21,726
Never married	8	6	98,582	103,688	−5,106
n	534	695	534	695	

The results presented in Figure 9.1 show that marital status is obviously important for the economic situation of older adults. This is underscored when disposable household income is calculated by gender and marital status (Table 9.1).

Generally women have a lower disposable income (median) than men. The difference overall is slightly more than SEK27,000 per year, or about SEK1,800 a month. Differences in equivalent disposable income are smaller among married/cohabiting couples, but here too women have a lower disposable income than men. This slightly surprising finding may be explained by age differences between men and women in most marriages. In general men are married to younger women; younger women have on average been in paid employment for longer than older married women. This means that younger women on average will have higher earnings–related supplementary pensions and thereby higher incomes than older women. Women, on the other hand, tend to be married to older men who are likely to have somewhat lower pensions than men of their own age or younger. All in all, then, being married to a younger woman (which most men are) gives rise to a higher disposable income for married men.

When we turn to single households we find much more pronounced gender differences in economic resources. The disparity in household income is over SEK20,000 per year between widowed and divorced men and women. Even if older men clearly have lower incomes when they are widowed or divorced, the differences between them and married or cohabiting men is much smaller than the corresponding difference among women.

By contrast, men who have never married have a lower income standard than their female counterparts. It is reasonable to believe that this is a result of earlier labour force participation. Men who never marry are traditionally more likely than other men to be socially and educationally disadvantaged, which in turn will affect their lifetime incomes and thereby their pensions. Women who have never married, on the other hand, are more likely than married women to have been in highly qualified jobs (Arber et al, 2003). Our data also show that these men, on average, have 7.2 years of schooling compared to 8.3 years for men who are or have been married. The corresponding figures for women are 9.1 and 7.7 years respectively. Our conclusion is therefore that the differences in the level of education of men and women in different marital status groups, and the differences in types of jobs and lifetime incomes that these educational differences imply, explain the reversed income difference between men and women who have never married. These women over 65 are a relatively advantaged group in terms of income compared with other women, while the opposite is the case for men who have never married.

Another dimension of economic resources is economic security, in the following defined as the lack of a cash margin. This indicator is based on a question that reads: 'If a situation suddenly arose in which you had to come up with SEK12,000 within a week, could you manage it?'. Those unable to produce a sum of this size, including those who would have to take a loan to obtain it, were regarded as lacking a cash margin. Being unable to raise a cash margin implies a certain degree of financial insecurity and limits a person's ability to obtain capital goods or manage a sudden economic crisis. This indicator reflects a different dimension of economic resources than disposable income, since it also takes wealth, savings and consumption into account. Whether the person has access to a cash margin is an indicator of economic security that is not necessarily linked to present income only. The correlation between these two indicators of economical resources is therefore modest among older adults in Sweden; Spearman's Rho is 0.24. We do nevertheless also find gender differences here. While nearly 17% of all older adults lack a cash margin, this is the case for about 20% of older women but only 13% of older men.

Table 9.2 presents the results of a logistic regression analysis. When we adjust for differences in age we still find a clearly elevated risk of a lack of economic security among women (OR = 1.74). Although women are more likely to lack a cash margin, their disadvantage in this case can to a substantial degree be explained by marital status. Thus, when gender differences in marital status are taken into account, women's higher risk of not having a cash margin is reduced to 1.43.

The OR of having no cash margin is much higher among the unmarried than among married couples. Seven out of 10 of those lacking a cash margin have never been married, or are divorced or widowed, with the widowed seeming to be in a better position than the divorced and the never married (model 2). Further, no significant interaction between gender and marital status was found; instead the findings are surprisingly similar for men and women (model 3). Among both men and women the divorced appear to have the largest risk of lacking an economic buffer. Although the elevated risk of having no cash margin among widowers has a confidence interval that includes 1, the point estimate is not significantly lower than that for widows.

Table 9.2: Odds ratios (OR) for lacking a cash margin by gender and marital status

	Model 1	Model 2	Model 3	
			Men	**Women**
	OR (95% CI)	**OR (95% CI)**	**OR (95% CI)**	**OR (95% CI)**
Gender				
Men	1.00	1.00		
Women	1.74 (1.3-2.4)	1.43 (1.0-2.0)		
Marital status				
Married		1.00	1.00	1.00
Widowed		2.18 (1.5-3.3)	1.75 (0.9-3.6)	2.31 (1.4-3.8)
Divorced		4.35 (2.6-7.2)	4.82 (2.2-10.5)	4.14 (2.2-8.0)
Never married		3.49 (2.0-6.1)	3.80 (1.7-8.3)	3.22 (1.5-7.1)
n	1,229	1,229	1,229	

Model 1 and model 2, adjusted for age group

Model 3, combined analyses adjusted for age group and interaction between gender and marital status

It is fairly uncommon both to have a low income and to lack a cash margin, as is indicated by the low correlation reported above. Nevertheless, here too there is a gender difference; almost 5% of older adults have a low income and lack a cash margin, but 70% of this group are women.

Thus, when it comes to economic resources, married people have a great advantage over unmarried people (including never married, divorced, and widowed). This is true for women as well as for men, and for incomes as well as for economic security in terms of the ability to raise a substantial amount of money. However, there are also differences in economic resources between men and women within each marital status. While these differences are small among married men and women, they are substantial among widowed and divorced people. There are effectively larger differences in disposable income between married and unmarried women than between married and unmarried men.

When interpreting the importance of these gender differences it is important to consider the large differences in marital status between older men and women. Whereas two out of three men over 65 years are married, only two out of five women are (see Table 9.1). Official statistics show that at the age of 80 this pattern is even clearer; 64% of men are married while only 31% of women are (Statistics Sweden, 2004). This, in turn, indicates that older women spend more years alone than men of their age, and in addition they tend to have smaller economic resources during these years. This raises the issue of what implications this has for other aspects of life, for example health and functional ability.

Health and functional ability

In Sweden, as in most countries, women have a higher life expectancy than men. In 2003 life expectancy at birth was 77.9 for men and 82.4 for women (Statistics Sweden, 2004). In recent decades men have had a more rapid increase in life expectancy than women. Life expectancy after the age of 65 increased by 1.3 years for women and 2.3 years for men during the period 1990-2003 (Figure 9.2). Over the same period, life expectancy after the age of 75 also increased more for men (0.8 years) than for women (0.5 years). The increase in longevity is to a large degree a result of falling mortality rates in coronary heart disease – the over-all mortality risk fell by 40% between 1987 and 2003 (NBHW, 2005a). These changes may be attributed to changes in smoking rates and lowered lipid levels, as well as improved treatments for and rehabilitations from chronic illnesses. The latter interpretation is supported by the fact that mortality has decreased more rapidly than have incidence rates (NBHW, 2005a).

There is now plenty of evidence showing that inequalities in life expectancy by socioeconomic status exist. Generally, individuals with a lower socioeconomic position die earlier than individuals with a higher socioeconomic position, and therefore also have a shorter life expectancy. This relationship has been observed for many European countries, including Sweden (Mackenbach et al, 1997;

Figure 9.2: Life expectancy at age 65 (1990-2003)

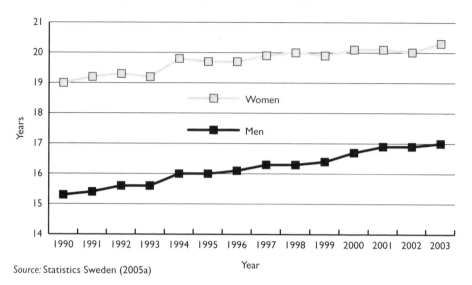

Source: Statistics Sweden (2005a)

Statistics Sweden, 2004), and it is found also for older adults (Lundberg and Kåreholt, 1996; Huisman et al, 2004, 2005).

Another well-established fact is that marital status in adulthood as well as among older adults is strongly associated with life expectancy. Married people can expect to live more years than unmarried people, a pattern that is valid for both men and women. In Sweden in 2003, married men could expect to live almost three years longer after 65 than widowers, and more than 4.1 years longer than never married men (Figure 9.3). Corresponding figures for women were 2.2 and

Figure 9.3: Life expectancy at age 65 by gender and marital status (2003)

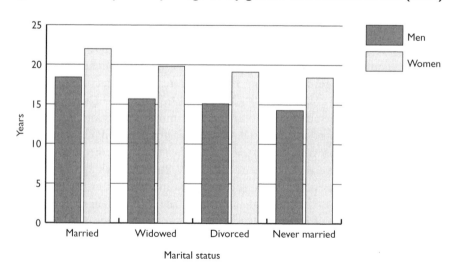

Source: Statistics Sweden (2004)

3.6 years (Statistics Sweden, 2004). More recently, research has also shown that over the past two decades the relative mortality differences between marital status groups have increased. This development is notable in several western and northern European countries and is due to a sharp decline in mortality among married couples (Valkonen et al, 2004).

As pointed out in Chapter One mortality data do not reflect the burden of ill health. There are health problems that cause much pain and suffering and reduce the ability to lead an independent life. Health problems also give rise to costs for treatment and care (Lahelma, 2001). There is ample evidence to show that health inequalities by gender, socioeconomic position and marital relationship persist into later life. In general women report more ill health than men, but the health disparity between men and women varies with different health outcomes (Macintyre et al, 1996; Fratiglioni et al, 1997; Arber and Cooper, 1999; Lahelma et al, 1999). Further, those with working-class occupations are more likely to suffer ill health and disability in later life than non-manual workers (Dahl and Birkelund, 1997; Arber and Cooper, 1999; Avlund et al, 2003; Huisman et al, 2003). Men and retired non-manual workers demonstrated a better health status than women and retired manual workers, both in terms of self-reported health and physical performance tests, also when aged over 75 (Thorslund et al, 1993, 2004; Thorslund and Lundberg, 1994). Moreover, socioeconomic inequalities measured by income are found to be related to health among older people in Sweden. Older adults with a high income are healthier than others when gender and age are adjusted for (Lundberg and Thorslund, 1996b).

Marital status has also been shown to be important for health and functional abilities in older age groups. In general, married people have the best health, followed by the never married and then the divorced, although a fairly weak or reversed relationship between marriage and health among older adults has been reported (Goldman et al, 1995; Murphy et al, 1997; Grundy and Sloggett, 2003). Furthermore, Arber (2004) found that there was little difference among men according to marital status, while all marital status groups of women were more likely to have severely impaired health than married men.

In the following we will further explore the inter-relationships between gender, marital status, economic resources and health in old age. Two measures related to health and functional ability are studied, namely mobility limitations and poor self-rated health (SRH). Functional ability is an important indicator of health in old age as it conveys information about the consequences of chronic diseases, that is, how impairments and functional limitations influence daily activities (Verbrugge and Jette, 1994). Impaired mobility can be regarded as a functional limitation, because it affects independent living. Self-reported mobility problems, as used in the following analyses, have been found to be strongly related to mobility assessed by performance tests (for example, Sayers et al, 2004). Self-rated health is dichotomised into 'poor' and 'in between good and poor' on the one hand and 'good' on the other. A section of the sample (82 people) was interviewed through proxies, usually a relative. Since proxy interviews are carried

Table 9.3: Odds ratios (OR) for mobility limitations and SRH less than good by gender and income groups

	Mobility limitations			SRH less than good		
	Model 1	Model 2	Model 3	Model 1	Model 2	Model 3
	OR (95% CI)	OR (95% CI)	OR (95% CI)	OR (95% CI)	OR (95% CI)	OR (95% CI)
Gender						
Men	1.00	1.00	1.00	1.00	1.00	1.00
Women	1.78 (1.4-2.3)	1.59 (1.2-2.1)	1.56 (1.2-2.0)	1.40 (1.1-1.8)	1.22 (1.0-1.6)	1.21 (0.9-1.5)
Income groups (SEK)						
<75,000		1.98 (1.1-3.5)	1.70 (1.0-3.0)		1.67 (1.0-2.8)	1.55 (0.9-2.6)
75,000-100,000		2.18 (1.4-3.3)	1.87 (1.2-2.9)		3.15 (2.1-4.7)	2.94 (2.0-4.4)
100,000-125,000		2.26 (1.5-3.5)	2.07 (1.3-3.2)		2.30 (1.5-3.4)	2.21 (1.5-3.3)
125,000-150,000		1.56 (1.0-2.5)	1.48 (0.9-2.4)		1.61 (1.1-2.5)	1.57 (1.0-2.4)
150,000-175,000		0.71 (0.4-1.3)	0.71 (0.4-1.3)		1.05 (0.6-1.7)	1.05 (0.7-1.7)
175,000+		1.00	1.00		1.00	1.00
Cash margin						
Yes			1.00			1.00
No			2.04 (1.5-2.9)			1.37 (1.0-1.9)
n	1,220	1,220	1,220	1,222	1,222	1,222

Note: All models adjusted for age group.

out when the subject is too ill to be interviewed in person, these subjects have all been categorised as having poor SRH.

The left-hand panel of Table 9.3 shows the OR for men and women of having mobility limitations, and what happens to the gender difference when income and cash margin are introduced to the model. As expected, model 1 shows that women have a higher risk of mobility limitations than men, also when age is controlled for.

In contrast to analyses of income and health generally (see Chapter Seven), we do not find a curvilinear relation between income and mobility limitations (model 2). Instead it appears that older adults with an annual disposable income of less than SEK150,000 have significantly higher levels of mobility limitation than those with higher incomes when gender and age are controlled for. However, only a small part of the gender difference in mobility limitations appears to be linked to gender differences in disposable income. The OR for women is reduced from 1.78 to 1.59. There is no statistically significant interaction between gender and income, meaning that the relation between income level and mobility is similar for women and men.

Those who do not have a cash margin have double the odds of having mobility limitations, even when age, gender and income are adjusted for. This pattern is found among both women and men. The effect of income, on the other hand, becomes diluted when cash margin is added to the model.

The analyses of gender, economic resources and self-reported health produce somewhat different results. To begin with, the gender difference in SRH is less pronounced, and a fair amount of this difference can be attributed to income differences. Income is also related to SRH in the curvilinear way that one might expect from analyses of younger people. Although lack of a cash margin is linked to poor health, this relation is much weaker. These differences aside, there are also some fundamental similarities; being a woman, having a lower income and lacking a cash margin increases the risk of poor SRH. Again, there is no interaction effect between gender and income.

Our analyses show that both a good income and access to a cash margin are of importance for health and functional ability among older adults, but is a cash margin equally important for health in both high and low-income groups? In order to analyse this, the data was stratified according to income group. Our result indicates (Figure 9.4) that access to a cash margin is most important among those with an annual equivalent disposable income of less than SEK150,000. It also seems that having or not having a cash margin is of greater significance for mobility limitations than for SRH.

Having examined gender inequalities in health and mobility among older adults and to what extent economic resources contribute to these inequalities, we next added marital status to the picture. First, we focus on the extent to which health and mobility limitations are related to marital status, and whether differences in marital status can explain gender differences in health. The results

Figure 9.4: Odds ratios (OR) for mobility limitations and SRH less than good by cash margin and annual income

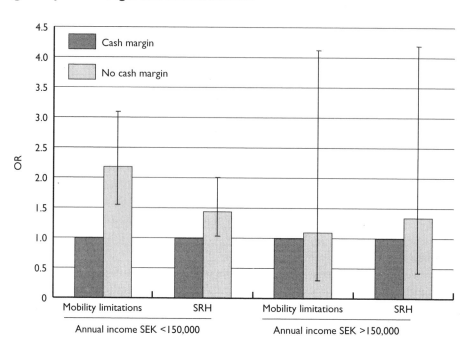

shown in Table 9.4, model 1 indicate that divorcees have significantly higher levels of mobility limitations than married people when gender and age are controlled for. The OR for women is also somewhat lower than in model 1 in Table 9.3, indicating that a smaller part of the gender difference in mobility limitations is due to differences in marital status. This finding is due to the fact that the main gender difference in marital status is in the proportion of widows and married, while the health differences between these groups are small.

When one performs an analysis stratified by gender (model 2) it also becomes evident that the main effects of marital status do not represent the patterns among men and women particularly well. Differences in mobility limitations by marital status are more pronounced among men than among women. Most strikingly, widowed women are not at all more prone to limited mobility, while widowers have an OR of 2.17. Among divorced women and men, on the other hand, the OR are fairly similar.

Secondly, we address the issue of the role of economic resources for the differences in mobility limitations between marital statuses for men and for women. As seen earlier, both equivalent disposable income and access to a cash margin have independent effects on health outcomes among women and men alike. Adding these indicators to the model also lowers the OR for single men and women (Table 9.4, model 3). Two substantial findings can be noted here. Firstly, much of the high risk of mobility limitations among divorced men and women

Table 9.4: Odds ratios (OR) for mobility limitations and SRH less than good by gender and marital status

	Model 1	Model 2		Model 3	
	All	Men	Women	Men	Women
	OR (95% CI)	OR (95% CI)	OR (95% CI)	OR (95% CI)	OR (95% CI)
(a) Mobility limitations					
Gender					
Men	1.00				
Women	1.66 (1.3-2.2)				
Marital status					
Married	1.00	1.00	1.00	1.00	1.00
Widowed	1.25 (0.9-1.7)	2.17 (1.3-3.6)	0.94 (0.6-1.4)	2.02 (1.2-3.4)	0.77 (0.5-1.2)
Divorced	2.05 (1.3-3.2)	2.10 (1.0-4.4)	1.89 (1.0-3.4)	1.56 (0.7-3.3)	1.26 (0.7-2.3)
Never married	1.21 (0.7-2.0)	1.43 (0.7-2.9)	0.98 (0.5-2.0)	1.00 (0.5-2.1)	0.76 (0.4-1.6)
n	1,220	1,220		1,220	
(b) SRH less than good					
Gender					
Men	1.00				
Women	1.35 (1.1-1.7)				
Marital status					
Married	1.00	1.00	1.00	1.00	1.00
Widowed	1.13 (0.8-1.5)	1.37 (0.8-2.3)	0.98 (0.7-1.4)	1.30 (0.8-2.2)	0.83 (0.6-1.2)
Divorced	1.56 (1.0-2.4)	1.22 (0.6-2.4)	1.76 (1.0-3.2)	0.94 (0.5-1.9)	1.17 (0.6-2.2)
Never married	1.24 (0.8-2.0)	2.54 (1.3-5.0)	0.57 (0.3-1.1)	1.95 (1.0-3.9)	0.47 (0.2-0.9)
n	1,219	1,219		1,219	

Model 1, adjusted for age group

Model 2, combined analyses, adjusted for age group and interaction between gender and marital status

Model 3, combined analyses, adjusted for age group, interaction between gender and marital status and economic resources

is due to the fact that they have poorer economic resources than married people of the same sex. Secondly, the elevated risk among widowers is not due to their economic situation.

If we shift focus to poor SRH we find a similar general pattern, although the OR are generally lower. Not much of the gender difference in SRH is due to differences in marital status, and when we look at main effects (model 1) it is the divorced who have a clearly higher illness risk. According to the gender-specific analysis in model 2, however, it appears that men who never married are the group with the highest risk, especially when compared with their female counterparts. Model 3 shows again that controlling for economic resources does reveal some effects. The health disadvantage of the divorced older adults, compared to married people, is partly a result of divorced men and women having poorer economic resources. Also worth noting is the fact that women who have never married report better SRH than married women when economic resources are adjusted for.

If the age-adjusted analyses are carried out by marital status group rather than by gender (not shown), we find that married women report more health problems than married men, even when economic resources are adjusted for. Among unmarried people there are no significant gender differences in mobility limitations or poor SRH. These findings do not change when economic resources are adjusted for.

Conclusion

Marital status and gender inequalities in old age

People over retirement age are sometimes regarded as a homogenous group of 'older people'. This is of course not the case; the diversity within this group is indeed substantial, not only on the basis of gender, socioeconomic status and other sociodemographic structures but also in terms of age and cohort membership. Inequalities at advanced age may therefore reflect both the results of the aging process as such and the accumulation of advantages or disadvantages across the life course.

The birth cohorts under study in this chapter were born between 1903 and 1935 and have, probably to a greater extent than other cohorts living today, experienced great societal developments and the growth of the welfare state. Welfare benefits such as the guarantee pension and health and old age care services are important resources for most older adults' lives. Even those who are not in immediate need of these services may regard them as an important insurance for future needs. Furthermore, health and old age care services can also be regarded as important resources for the spouse and children of people in need of regular or temporary care. Thus, well functioning welfare is important not only for the person in need but also for those around him or her.

However, since the late 1980s old age care has become characterised by prioritisation and the concentration of help and care to a smaller group of older people with extensive help needs. Old age care has thereby been transformed into a more medical form of care while help of a more domestic kind and less intensive care are left to family members and the market (Palme et al, 2003; Szebehely, 2005). These changes have been described as an informalisation and marketisation of municipal care and are unevenly distributed in terms of both gender and class (for a discussion see Szebehely, 2000, 2005).

These changes shape the structural conditions against which our analyses should be read. Another structural condition of importance for our analyses is the age difference between spouses, that is, the fact that at any given age the interviewee's spouse is on average younger if our interviewee is a man, but older if the interviewee is a woman. Since men die younger, women are more likely to become widows and have to deal with everyday life alone. For older men the situation is quite the opposite.

We have focused on economic and health resources, on how these resources are linked to marital status and in what way they differ between men and women. We have tried to gain a better understanding of gender inequalities in health and mobility by simultaneously analysing the importance of marital status, with economic resources as a possible mediating factor.

Our results show that both men and women have better economic resources when married. The differences between married and single people are, however, larger among women. This suggests that being married is beneficial for economic wellbeing for both men and women but especially for women. Since women are likely to spend more years alone they also experience more years living at a low economic standard. For women, then, widowhood may over and above the grief of a lost spouse lead to reduction in economic standard.

Men of all marital statuses have higher disposable incomes than women, with one exception – men who have never married have a lower income standard than their female counterparts. This may be linked to the fact that women who have never married have more years of schooling than both married women and men who have never married. We argue that the explanation for the divergent income pattern could be a result of different patterns not only in schooling, but also in terms of labour force participation and the types of job held during working life. In other words, never to have married is likely to reflect quite different life careers for women and men in these cohorts. For women of these generations it was often impossible to combine an occupational career with a family; among men, on the other hand, not being married may rather reflect a certain degree of marginalisation, sometimes early on in life (see, for example, Modin, 2003).

Despite the fact that women in general outlive men they more often report health problems, and, according to our results, older women have poorer health than men in the same age groups. Although there is a clear gender difference in poor SRH, differences in mobility limitations are steeper. There are also health differences between marital status groups, but these differences are also patterned by gender. And although gender inequalities vary depending on marital status, married women report more health problems than married men. While mobility limitations and poorer health are more common among divorced people than married people of both sexes, widowers and men who have never married experience more ill health and mobility limitations, while this is not the case among their female counterparts. Thus, marriage has a health protecting effect for older men. A recent British study by Grundy and Sloggett (2003) also found no health advantage for married older women and a possible advantage of never having married for women.

The gender differences among widowed people also indicate that the advantage for health of being married is greater for older men than for older women. Since women are usually younger than their spouses, they reach the age at which illnesses and dependency are more usual after their spouses. Moreover, women traditionally take responsibility for caring for their dependent spouses. Widowhood might therefore actually mean a reduction in caring responsibilities. Furthermore, the lack of health advantage for married older women is a fairly unexpected finding since our data also includes women living in institutions, who as a rule are in poorer health than women still living in their own homes.

Whereas economic resources are linked to health and functional ability among both older and younger adults, the shape of this relationship is different for the two types of outcome. For mobility limitations there is a threshold relationship, with those below a yearly disposable income of SEK150,000 (corresponding to 74% of all those 65+) having an increased risk. In addition, lack of a cash margin raises the risk even further. For SRH, on the other hand, the relationship is more curvilinear, and there is a clearly weaker independent effect of not having a cash margin. The reasons for this difference are unclear, although they might be related to the different content of the two measures; SRH reflects a wider range of health problems, including perhaps also life satisfaction, while mobility limitations only reflects more specific mobility problems. It might also reflect different timeframes, with mobility limitations reflecting a lifetime accumulation of absolute health risks and SRH reflecting a person's present situation vis-à-vis that of other older adults.

While equivalent disposable household income and access to a cash margin have independent impacts on health outcomes for both women and men, they do not account for much of the gender differences in health and mobility. Similarly, the association between marital status and the two health outcomes under study remains fairly unchanged when economic resources are controlled for. Only the higher risk of poorer health among divorced people is partly due to the fact that they have poorer economic resources than married people.

In conclusion, the findings presented in this chapter, in line with earlier studies, demonstrate that marriage determines living conditions in later life differently for men and women. In general terms, the empirical evidence suggests that men benefit more from marriage than women, while women benefit more than men in terms of economic resources. And although single older women are generally worse off economically, this is not reflected in their health and functional abilities. While economic resources are important for health, other factors are therefore more central for preserving health and functional abilities in old age.

TEN

Health inequalities and welfare resources: findings and forecasts

Johan Fritzell, Carin Lennartsson and Olle Lundberg

Introduction

In this book we have analysed and discussed different forms of health inequalities, their size and shape, how they have changed over time, and how they are portrayed across various parts of the life course. We have also analysed a number of social determinants of health and how these may generate and sustain health inequalities. In doing this, we took Scandinavian welfare research as our point of departure in order to establish a conceptual framework of "command over resources ... by means of which the individual can control and consciously direct her conditions of life" (Johansson, 1970, p 25). Resources central to health include work and working conditions, income and economic resources, family and social relations, all of which are brought into the analysis in several of the chapters.

The analyses in the book also rest on the welfare research tradition, in that we employ databases designed for the purpose of describing and analysing the distribution and development of welfare problems. Our main data source is the Swedish Level-of-Living Survey (LNU), but we also use Statistics Sweden's yearly Survey of Living Conditions (ULF) as well as amendments and extensions of these two databases that incorporate schoolchildren and the oldest old. Taken together, these data have enabled us to study social determinants of health over time, as well as to look across the life course from the age of nine to 99.

The general context for our analyses of health and inequalities is the Swedish welfare state. Changes in health and health inequalities are also discussed against the background of changes in welfare state institutions. Although the Swedish case may be seen as an 'ideal type' of what is known as the Scandinavian welfare state model, it is also likely that the crucial determinants of ill health, and how these are systematically related to social position in market societies, will share basic characteristics across countries. While different welfare state arrangements are likely to modify the processes linking social position with health outcomes (see below), these processes themselves will be similar in different types of welfare state. Although Sweden may stand out as an exception in terms of the ambitions of the welfare state and the strength of the economic and welfare state crisis experienced during the 1990s, our findings regarding mechanisms are therefore also applicable to other societies.

While many social determinants can be seen as general, influencing people's health and living conditions irrespective of time and place, we make one further claim. The welfare state may be of importance in three ways: first, by influencing the prevalence of social and other determinants of health; second, by influencing the way in which these explanatory risk factors are distributed across social strata; and third, by acting as a buffer by breaking the links between the determinants and their influence on health. In this concluding chapter we will summarise the general findings of the book as a whole, as well as relate these findings to the present discussion about health and inequalities. We will also discuss some of the more general findings from the perspective of comparative welfare state analysis.

In terms of exploring the size of, or changes in, health inequalities, the two dimensions that dominate in this book are socioeconomic and gender inequalities. We study socioeconomic inequalities as class differentials (Chapters Two and Four) and as health differentials by income (Chapters Seven and Nine). Gender inequalities are touched on in most chapters but are the focus of particular attention in Chapter Three. Both class and gender differences are studied from a time perspective. Some chapters concentrate on specific age groups, others explore how gender or class differences evolve over time or over the life course. In addition to a discussion about class and gender inequalities, we also comment on the general findings regarding age and country of birth.

In terms of determinants or mediating factors some chapters are more directly linked to specific debates in the international research community, making use of middle-range theories and testing their empirical validity. Our main ambition in these chapters is not so much to describe these inequalities but rather the more ambitious aim of trying to understand them. This is the case in Chapters Five, Six, Seven, Eight and Nine, which discuss and empirically test, for example, the importance of sense of coherence, the psychosocial work environment (both for adults and schoolchildren), relative deprivation and social capital. These chapters thereby not only investigate whether such theoretical constructs might be of importance for health status, but also to what extent they are important when we try to explain the gradient by class or gender.

Socioeconomic inequalities: changes over time and over the life course

As we mentioned initially in this book, people's position in the social structure is most often discussed and studied from the perspective of social class. The class one belongs to is of fundamental importance in the sense that it is linked to certain rewards and resources. These can be monetary or more immaterial in nature, for example status, power or autonomy, which in turn might be of importance for other types of resources, including economic resources. Not surprisingly then, class differences are found in virtually all spheres of life. Their relation with health, we would argue, is likely to be an effect of both material and immaterial resources linked to class position.

The more or less universal nature of class or socioeconomic inequalities has recently been debated in the health inequality literature in relation to the discussion of 'fundamental causes' (Link and Phelan, 1995; Phelan et al, 2004). In his discussion of research strategies, Lieberson (1985) suggested a distinction between basic and superficial causes. He argued that most causes explored, in social sciences at least, are superficial in the sense that they are merely 'symptoms' of the basic causes. Consequently, elimination of a superficial cause will not fundamentally alter the basic relation, even in cases where the influence of a superficial cause is strong. While we have not been aiming to prove the accuracy of this proposition it is a fact that class inequalities in most of the health outcomes we have presented were remarkably stable from the late 1960s up until the new millennium, despite a vast number of societal and individually related changes over the same period.

What has not radically changed, of course, is the fact that those in higher social strata generally have more *command over resources*, which is indeed also the key concept in the welfare approach adopted here. Interestingly enough this coincides extremely well with the position taken by Link and Phelan (1995) when they claim that the reason for socioeconomic inequalities being fundamental, persistent, and reproductive is that they are linked to access to resources. Their definition of resources thus broadly concurs with our definition in Chapter One.

This is not to say that class inequalities are always present with respect to specific diseases, specific periods of the life course or that they are constant across time. Indeed, this book contains several indications of where the opposite is the case. Most strikingly, but generally consistent with other research findings, Modin and Östberg (Chapter Six) note that class inequalities in ill health are virtually non-existent among Swedish children aged 9-18. Similarly, the life course perspective taken by Fritzell (Chapter Four) indicates that class inequalities do indeed vary in different stages of life, first by increasing and then possibly decreasing somewhere around retirement age. This does not mean that class inequalities vanish completely in old ages. As shown by Lennartsson and Lundberg (Chapter Nine) substantial socioeconomic differences do indeed exist among the oldest in Sweden, although the stratification variable used here is income.

By and large, when we compare the Sweden of the late 1960s with the Sweden of 2000 we find class inequalities to be fairly stable – or at least we find no tendency towards a reduction in class differences. In line with the idea of accumulation of health risks over the life course, our findings suggest that the total impact of class is greater than cross-sectional analyses might suggest. Thus, although we do find that class of origin has become less important in more recent birth cohorts (Chapter Four), our main conclusion is that social class remains an important determinant of health in modern societies.

Gender differences over time and in different phases of life

Gender differences in the risk of ill health seem to exist across the whole life span. As shown by Modin and Östberg (Chapter Six) there are considerable gender gaps in psychosomatic complaints and psychological wellbeing during childhood and adolescence, while class differentials are negligible in these age groups (Östberg et al, 2006). Although children's psychosocial work environment at school, as measured by the demand–control–support model, is of great importance per se, these conditions do not explain the gender gap in wellbeing as such.

We also find substantial gender differentials at the other end of the life cycle. Mobility limitations are much more common among older women than among men of the same age. Thus, Lennartsson and Lundberg (Chapter Nine) demonstrate that these differentials are in part related to economic resources, as well as to a complex interrelation between age at marriage, marital status and average life expectancy.

While women have a higher life expectancy than men, our analyses indicate that women experience more ill health than men for all health indicators studied. Hemström, Krantz and Roos (Chapter Three) scrutinise in detail gender differences and changes therein for two of our most widely used indices of ill health, namely musculoskeletal pain and psychological distress, over a 32-year period. These are indicators that cover the vast majority of all sickness leave on the Swedish labour market. Women report more musculoskeletal pain than men and this difference has increased. Women also have a higher risk of psychological distress, although this excess risk is fairly stable over time.

Given Sweden's reputation with regard to gender equality these findings are perhaps surprising. Seen over the whole period covered in our study, the increase in female labour market attachment is one of the greatest transitions in Swedish society. In this respect, Sweden is a leader in what today is an international trend. This dramatic change has in many ways been facilitated by political reforms, especially with regard to childcare, although other welfare services and tax reforms have also contributed to this change. In most international comparisons Sweden is singled out as the most gender equal country in the world. Our finding of no decrease in gender differences in ill health, and even of a widening of the gender gap in musculoskeletal pain, is thus quite intriguing. Moreover, although overall life expectancy has increased, improvements for women have been smaller than for men. Indeed, among women in lower social strata hardly any improvement in life expectancy can be detected.

How are we, then, to interpret these findings? First, we need to consider the deep recession that hit Sweden in the early 1990s: most of the widening of gender inequalities in health occurred in the 1990s. Sweden has, like most countries, a gender-segregated labour market in which a large share of women work in the public sector, and it was here in particular that a number of efficiency-driven organisational changes took place in the mid-1990s. These took the form of staff cutbacks as well as rising workload with fixed resources. As discussed by Toivanen (Chapter Five), numerous studies have also shown that psychosocial working conditions worsened in the 1990s, especially in female-dominated workplaces. The most dramatic effect of the recession, however, was the change in employment rates. Although Sweden has a reputation of having a very high female labour force participation rate it actually fell from an all-time high in 1990 of 81% to below 70% in 1996-98, after which it has increased slightly again (72% in 2004). Since male labour force participation rates fell in a similar way, gender differences in this respect are very similar before and after the 1990s. It is thus important also to interpret the remaining gender inequalities in health in light of this massive decrease in paid employment, partly driven by the cuts made in the welfare state during and after the recession, and not only in relation to the political efforts to increase gender equality in the first place.

Second, although women's position and autonomy is probably better in Sweden than in most other countries, there are still gender inequalities in working hours, wages, career opportunities and household division of labour that may play a role in explaining health differences. Third, even if diminishing gender inequalities in working and family life failed to eliminate gender differentials in ill health, we should not stop striving for a gender equal society. As discussed by Mackenbach (2005b), one sometimes has to balance public health with the value of individual autonomy. Indeed, the struggle for individual autonomy has often been seen as a key to improving women's position in society (Orloff, 1993). Consequently, political reforms aiming to increase gender equality are important per se, regardless of their impact on health.

Age – not merely a confounder

As we see in Chapter Two, there has been a general change in the age profile of ill health. More specifically, health and functional abilities have improved in the older age groups included in the analysis (66-75; for some health indicators 56-75), while the age group 19-49 has experienced deteriorating health. Accordingly, the almost exponential increase in poor health with increasing age that prevailed at the end of the 1960s has turned into a much flatter slope 30 years later.

This change is, we would argue, the result of two different processes. In the older age groups, later born cohorts have entered old age in better health, not least due to improvements in living conditions and life chances throughout life. As discussed in Chapter Two, the poor development of health in younger age groups may be explained by poorer living conditions and greater stress and anxiety about the future.

Younger age groups have indeed been experiencing stagnating or even deteriorating living conditions and life chances since 1980 in both relative and absolute terms. For example, the real incomes for those aged below 30 stagnated in the 1980s and fell in the 1990s, and in relation to average incomes those aged under 50 have been lagging behind for the past 25 years (Fritzell and Lundberg,

1994; Palme et al, 2003). This may be linked to the fact that although a higher proportion of people are going on to higher education, the share of those who are overqualified for their jobs has also increased. This, in turn, is likely to reduce the economic returns on education (le Grand et al, 2004). At the same time, youth unemployment rates have continued to remain high (Statistics Sweden, 2005c). Family formation has also been delayed, as indicated by the fact that the average age at first birth has risen by almost five years since 1970 to 29 in 2004.

Taken together, all these more specific changes in living conditions also seem to indicate, or in some cases even generate, a greater degree of uncertainty among young people regarding the future. Greater uncertainty or reduced predictability is in itself likely to give rise to stress and anxiety. In addition, it will increase the importance of making the 'right' decisions about education, occupational career and family formation, which in turn will also increase stress and anxiety. The fact that psychological distress has increased much more sharply than other types of health problem in younger age groups suggests that mechanisms of this kind are important. Given the strong and (so far) stable relation between reported anxiety and much more severe forms of poor mental health (Ringbäck Weitoft and Rosén, 2005), these recent trends may represent a serious and growing public health problem for the future.

Differences by country of birth

We find substantial inequalities in health between people born in Sweden, people born in OECD countries and those born outside the OECD area, despite the fact that this categorisation by country of birth is very crude. Most typically, people born in poorer countries (non-OECD) often have poorer health than the other two groups, but this is not always the case. Immigrants from OECD countries also tend to have poorer health than people born in Sweden, although this finding is likely to be the result of poor health among the large group of Finns.

While immigrants in general, and refugees in particular, may be vulnerable due to poor conditions or experiences in their country of origin, including persecution, war, famine or torture, these groups are also disadvantaged in almost all spheres of life of importance to health when they come to Sweden. Furthermore, immigrants were hit more severely than other groups by the recession in the 1990s. In other words, their living conditions worsened much more than those of native Swedes (Fritzell and Lundberg, 2000b). Consequently, while some of the differences we found might be related to life course events before coming to Sweden, we firmly believe that present living conditions are highly relevant when trying to explain present health inequalities between people born in different countries. The importance of social factors was also highlighted by Rostila (Chapter Eight), who found that adjusting for different informal and formal social contacts substantially reduced the excess risk of ill health.

Our findings, by and large, reveal that health differentials between groups neither increased nor decreased over the longer time period covered by our data. However, this is not to say that the impact on population health has been stable. While in the late 1960s the group born in OECD countries, mostly Finns, was more than three times as large as the group born outside OECD, in 2000 the latter was almost twice as numerous as the former. In that respect the relatively stable excess risk represents an increasingly important public health problem.

Command over resources versus psychosocial or material explanations

A key question in the field of health inequalities research is how to explain the fact that such inequalities persist in wealthy societies. While there has been a great deal of consensus about the basic description of these inequalities, the mechanisms involved in generating inequalities have been highly debated. Two types of interpretation have dominated these debates. The first maintains that health inequalities are mainly generated by psychosocial factors such as people's relative standing causing poor health through stress mechanisms. The second basically suggests that differences in health risks are mainly caused directly by differences in actual living conditions (neo-material explanations). While both of these arguments have their merits, we would claim that it is wrong to present them as two opposite and mutually exclusive poles.

The psychosocial argument rests on the fact that health inequalities affect the whole population and are not only a problem of the poorest or most marginalised 5% (Marmot, 2004). On the basis of this observation, the argument for psychosocial mechanisms is that differences in health and mortality between richer and poorer in today's western societies are not due to differences in nutrition, shelter or poor sanitation; rather it is differences in status and relative income that affect health through various stress mechanisms.

In contrast, the neo-material argument claims that it is the direct and concrete health effects of poor material circumstances that are of importance, rather than any relative comparison with people who are better off. In effect, it is not psychosocial stress mechanisms that are important, but rather more proximal health risks linked to specific exposures related to poor living conditions. The difference is illustrated by Lynch and colleagues:

> Differences in neo-material conditions between first and economy class may produce health inequalities after a long flight. First class passengers get, among other advantages such as better food and service, more space and a wider, more comfortable seat that reclines into a bed. First class passengers arrive refreshed and rested, while many in economy arrive feeling a bit rough. Under a psychosocial interpretation, these health inequalities are due to negative emotions engendered by perceptions of relative disadvantage. Under a neo-material interpretation, people in economy have worse health because

> they sat in a cramped space and an uncomfortable seat, and they were
> not able to sleep. The fact that they can see the bigger seats as they
> walk off the plane is not the cause of poorer health. (Lynch et al,
> 2000, pp 1202-3)

The approach adopted in this book, in line with the Scandinavian welfare research tradition, is rather that *command over resources* by which we can control and consciously direct our conditions of life is of vital importance for health. These resources include both the material and the intangible. People higher up in the social structure have more command over resources, and are therefore more able to be in control and to act. They have, for example, a larger choice of where and how to live, and this larger scope of action also leads to a greater sense of control, which is further health enhancing. Having a low income will on the other hand reduce one's purchasing power and limit one's choices to cheaper food, cheaper housing, cheaper transportation and so on. This in turn is likely to affect health directly, through, for example less nutritious food and fewer hours of sleep. But it will *also* affect health by various stress-related processes driven by feelings of shame, anger, hopelessness and despair. And this idea is not even especially new; remember the causes of health inequalities as listed by Abraham Bäck: "… poverty, misery, lack of bread, anxiety and despair" (Bäck, 1765, p 7). Or, as Michael Marmot puts it, "… for people above a threshold of material well-being, another kind of well-being is central. Autonomy – how much control you have over your life – and the opportunities you have for full social engagement and participation are crucial for health, well-being and longevity. It is inequality in these that plays a big part in producing the social gradient in health" (Marmot, 2004, p 2).

One specific condition, therefore, may generate poor health both directly and through psychosocial mechanisms. This interpretation also helps us to understand why poorer people are affected harder; poor people have poorer health because they are more likely to be hit by a combination of the two mechanisms. Following the discussion in Chapter Seven, we would maintain that relative income is less important for health among the poor than among the rich, but that such relative effects nevertheless are likely to operate across the whole income range. The absolute effects of income, related directly to purchasing power, are likely to wear off as we move upwards in the income distribution. The combined effects of absolute and relative mechanisms may therefore explain the curvilinear relationship usually found between income and health.

Living conditions per se and the ways in which people understand and react to these conditions are not only additive, but may also interact with each other. As demonstrated by Toivanen in Chapter Five, a strong sense of coherence may modify the health consequences of both physical and psychological demands at work. Although this is not similar for men and women, these results further underline the importance of *combining* material and psychosocial explanations of health inequalities. Similarly, as shown by Rostila in Chapter Eight, the lack of social relations seems to be an important factor behind the increased risk of ill health among immigrants. As we have previously mentioned, immigrants tend also to have poorer material conditions. Again, this underlines the importance of combining different types of explanation.

Although the combination of these two explanations, combined under the concept of *command over resources*, can help us to better understand the mechanisms behind class inequalities in modern societies, the big question still remains: why do health inequalities persist even in Sweden at the magnitude demonstrated in this book? Does it mean that the welfare state project pursued for more than half a century has failed? We do not believe so, but an exhaustive answer to that important question would have to be based on comparative and historic analyses as well as the types of analyses undertaken here. The analyses presented in this book do, however, allow us to draw one conclusion regarding the welfare state. The economic crisis of the 1990s was the deepest recession experienced in Sweden since the 1930s. To some extent this crisis gave rise to poorer public health in general, yet by and large inequalities in health have not increased. This, we would argue, indicates that the welfare state was able to buffer the immediate impact of the crisis.

This is, of course, only an indication of the importance of welfare state institutions. Historical facts, like high rates of literacy or early implementation of maternal care, may still contribute to public health in Sweden. In addition, common features of the Nordic welfare state model, such as universalism, commitment to full employment and low poverty rates, are also likely to be important. Thus, while it is likely that the Nordic experience of welfare state policies have been important for public health and health inequalities, the basic social structures that generate differences in the amount of resources people command will remain. However, the Swedish case suggests that social policies have the potential to modify the relation between resources and health, and the degree to which they do so will literally affect the life chances of millions of people.

References

Åberg Yngwe, M., Lundberg, O. and Burström, B. (2006) 'On the importance of internalized consumption norms for ill-health', *Scandinavian Journal of Public Health*, vol 34, pp 76-82.

Åberg Yngwe, M., Fritzell, J., Burström, B. and Lundberg, O. (2005) 'Comparison or consumption? Distinguishing between different effects of income on health in Nordic welfare states', *Social Science & Medicine*, vol 61, pp 627-35.

Åberg Yngwe, M., Fritzell, J., Lundberg, O., Diderichsen, F. and Burström, B. (2003) 'Exploring relative deprivation: is social comparison a mechanism in the relation between income and health?', *Social Science & Medicine*, vol 57, pp 1463-73.

Abrahamsson, P. (1999) 'The welfare modelling business', *Social Policy & Administration*, vol 33, pp 394-415.

Agardh, E.E., Ahlbom, A., Andersson, T., Efendic, S., Grill, V., Hallqvist, J., Norman, A. and Ostenson, C.-G. (2003) 'Work stress and low sense of coherence is associated with type 2 diabetes in middle-aged Swedish women', *Diabetes Care*, vol 26, pp 719-24.

Ahlbom, A. and Alfredsson, L. (2005) 'Interaction: a word with two meanings creates confusion', *European Journal of Epidemiology*, vol 20, pp 563-4.

Aittomäki, A., Lahelma, E., Roos, E., Leino-Arjas, P. and Martikainen, P. (2005) 'Gender differences in the association of age with physical workload and functioning', *Occupational and Environmental Medicine*, vol 62, pp 95-100.

Åkerstedt, T. (2003) 'Återhämtning/sömn' ['Recuperation/sleep'], in T. Theorell (ed) *Psykosocal miljö och stress*, Lund: Studentlitteratur.

Albertsen, K., Nielsen, M.L. and Borg, V. (2001) 'The Danish psychosocial work environment and symptoms of stress: the main, mediating and moderating role of sense of coherence', *Work & Stress*, vol 15, pp 241-53.

Alcock, P., Glennerster, H., Oakley, A. and Sinfield, A. (eds) (2001) *Welfare and wellbeing: Richard Titmuss's contribution to social policy*, Bristol: The Policy Press.

Alwin, D. (1992) 'Aging, cohorts, and social change: an examination of the generational replacement model of social change', in H. Becker (ed) *Dynamics of cohort and generations research*, Amsterdam: Thesis Publicer, pp 53-95.

Andersson, L.-G., Erikson, R. and Wärneryd, B. (1981) 'Att beskriva den sociala strukturen. Utvärdering av 1974 års förslag till socio-ekonomisk indelning' ['Describing the social structure. A memo on the 1974 socio-economic classification'], *Statistisk Tidskrift*, pp 113-36.

Andersson, T., Alfredsson, L., Kallberg, H., Zdravkovic, S. and Ahlbom, A. (2005) 'Calculating measures of biological interaction', *European Journal of Epidemiology*, vol 20, pp 575-9.

Antonovsky, A. (1979) *Health, stress, and coping*, London: Jossey-Bass.

Antonovsky, A. (1987a) *Unraveling the mystery of health: How people manage stress and stay well*, San Francisco, CA: Jossey-Bass.

Antonovsky, A. (1987b) 'Health promoting factors at work: the sense of coherence', in R. Kalimo, M.A. El-Batawi and C.L. Cooper (eds) *Psychosocial factors at work and their relation to health*, Geneva: World Health Organisation, pp 153-67.

Antonovsky, A. (1991) 'The structural sources of salutogenic strengths', in C.L. Cooper and R. Payne (eds) *Personality and stress: Individual differences in the stress process*, Chichester: John Wiley & Sons, pp 67-104.

Antonovsky, A. (1993) 'The structure and properties of the sense of coherence scale', *Social Science & Medicine*, vol 36, pp 725-33.

Antonovsky, A., Sagy, S., Adler, I. and Visel, R. (1990) 'Attitudes toward retirement in an Israeli cohort', *International Journal of Aging and Human Development*, vol 31, pp 57-77.

Arber, S. (2004) 'Gender, marital status, and ageing: linking material, health, and social resources', *Journal of Aging Studies*, vol 18, pp 91-108.

Arber, S. and Cooper, H. (1999) 'Gender differences in health in later life: the new paradox?', *Social Science & Medicine*, vol 48, pp 61-76.

Arber, S. and Ginn, J. (1991) *Gender and later life: A sociological analysis of resources and constraints*, London: Sage Publications.

Arber, S. and Thomas, H. (2001) 'From women's health to a gender analysis of health', in W.C. Cockerham (ed) *The Blackwell companion to medical sociology*, Oxford: Blackwell Publishers, pp 94-113.

Arber, S., Price, D., Davidson, K. and Perren, K. (2003) 'Re-examining gender and marital status: material well-being and social involvement', in S. Arber, K. Davidson and J. Ginn (eds) *Gender and ageing: Changing roles and relationships*, Maidenhead: Open University Press.

Ariëns, G.A.M., van Mechelen, W., Bongers, P.M., Bouter, L.M. and van der Wal, G. (2001) 'Psychosocial risk factors for neck pain: a systematic review', *American Journal of Industrial Medicine*, vol 39, pp 180-93.

Aro, A.R., Nyberg, N., Absetz, P., Henriksson, M. and Lönnqvist, J. (2001) 'Depressive symptoms in middle-aged women are more strongly associated with physical health and social support than with socioeconomic factors', *Nordic Journal of Psychiatry*, vol 55, pp 191-8.

Aronsson, G., and Lindh, T. (2004) 'Långtidsfriskas arbetsvillkor. En populationsstudie' ['Work conditions among workers with good long term health. A population study'], *Arbete och hälsa*, vol 10, pp 1-21.

Artazcoz, L., Borrell, C. and Benach, J. (2001) 'Gender inequalities in health among workers: the relation with family demands', *Journal of Epidemiology and Community Health*, vol 55, pp 639-47.

Atkinson, T., Cantillon, B., Marlier, E. and Nolan, B. (2002) *Social indicators: The EU and social inclusion*, Oxford: Oxford University Press.

Avlund, K., Holstein, B.E., Osler, M., Damsgaard, M.T., Holm-Pedersen, P. and Rasmussen, N.K. (2003) 'Social position and health in old age: the relevance of different indicators of social position', *Scandinavian Journal of Public Health*, vol 31, pp 126-36.

Axelsson, C. (1992) *Hemmafrun som försvann: övergången till lönearbete bland gifta kvinnor i Sverige 1968-1981* [*The housewife that disappeared*], Stockholm: Swedish Institute for Social Research.

Bäck, A. (1765) *Tal om farsoter som mäst härja bland rikets allmoge* [*Speech on epidemics that lay waste among the country people of the realm*], Stockholm: Lars Salvius.

Bäckman, O. (2001) 'Med välfärdsstaten som arbetsgivare: arbetsmiljön och dess konsekvenser inom välfärdstjänsteområdet på 1990-talet' ['Employed by the welfare state: the working environment and its consequences in the welfare service sector in the 1990s'], in M. Szebehely (ed) *Välfärdstjänster i omvandling* [*Welfare services in transition*], (SOU) 2001:52, Stockholm: Fritzes.

Barker, D.J.P. (1998) *Mothers, babies and health in later life*, Edinburgh: Churchill Livingstone.

Baron, R.M. and Kenny, D.A. (1986) 'The moderator-mediator variable distinction in social psychological research: conceptual, strategic, and statistical considerations', *Journal of Personality and Social Psychology*, vol 51, pp 1173-82.

Belkic, K., Landsbergis, P., Schnall, P. and Baker, D. (2004) 'Is job strain a major source of cardiovascular disease risk?', *Scandinavian Journal of Work, Environment and Health*, vol 30, pp 85-128.

Bell, D. (1973) *The coming of post-industrial society. A venture in social forecasting*, New York, NY: Basic Books.

Ben-Shlomo, Y. and Kuh, D. (2002) 'A life course approach to chronic disease epidemiology: conceptual models, empirical challenges and interdisciplinary perspectives', *International Journal of Epidemiology*, vol 31, pp 285-93.

Berkley, K.J. (1997) 'Sex differences in pain', *Behavioral and Brain Sciences*, vol 20, pp 371-80.

Berkman, L. and Glass, T. (2000) 'Social integration, social networks, social support, and health', in L. Berkman and I. Kawaci (eds) *Social epidemiology*, New York, NY: Oxford University Press, pp 137-73.

Berkman, L.F. and Syme, S.L. (1979) 'Social networks, host resistance, and mortality: a nine-year follow-up study of Alameda county residents', *American Journal of Epidemiology*, vol 109, pp 186-204.

Berkman, L.F., Glass, T., Brissette, I. and Seeman, T.E. (2000) 'From social integration to health: Durkheim in the new millennium', *Social Science & Medicine*, vol 51, pp 843-57.

Bernard, B.P. (ed) (1997) *Musculoskeletal disorders and workplace factors. A critical review of epidemiologic evidence for work-related musculoskeletal disorders of the neck, upper extremity, and low back*, Cincinnati: NIOSH, US Department of Health and Human Services.

Berntsson, L.T. and Köhler, L. (2001) 'Long-term illness and psychosomatic complaints in children aged 2-17 years in the five Nordic countries. Comparison between 1984 and 1996', *European Journal of Public Health*, vol 11, pp 35-42.

Bingefors, K. and Isacson, D. (2004) 'Epidemiology, co-morbidity, and impact on health-related quality of life of self-reported headache and musculoskeletal pain – a gender perspective', *European Journal of Pain*, vol 8, pp 435-50.

Blaxter, M. (1989) *Health and lifestyles*, London: Tavistock/Routledge.

Blaxter, M. (2004) *Health*, Cambridge: Polity Press.

Boje, T. (1996) 'Welfare state models in comparative research: do the models describe reality?', in B. Greve (ed) *Comparative welfare systems: The Scandinavian model in a period of change*, Houndmills: Macmillan Press Ltd, pp 13-27.

Bolin, K., Lindgren, B., Lindström, M. and Nystedt, P. (2003) 'Investments in social capital – implications of social interactions for the production of health', *Social Science & Medicine*, vol 56, pp 2379-90.

Bongers, P.M., Kremer, A.M. and ter Laak, J. (2002) 'Are psychosocial factors, risk factors for symptoms and signs of the shoulder, elbow, or hand/wrist?: a review of the epidemiological literature', *American Journal of Industrial Medicine*, vol 41, pp 315-42.

Bourbonnais, R., Brisson, C., Moisan, J. and Vézina, M. (1996) 'Job strain and psychological distress in white-collar workers', *Scandinavian Journal of Work, Environment and Health*, vol 22, pp 139-45.

Bourbonnais, R., Comeau, M., Vezina, M. and Dion, G. (1998) 'Job strain, psychological distress, and burnout in nurses', *American Journal of Industrial Medicine*, vol 34, pp 20-8.

Bourdieu, P. (1986) 'The forms of capital', in J. G. Richardson (ed) *Handbook of theory and research for the sociology of education*, Westport, CT: Greenwood Press, pp 241-58.

Bovier, P., Chamot, E. and Perneger, T.V. (2004) 'Perceived stress, internal resources, and social support as determinants of mental health among young adults', *Quality of Life Research*, vol 13, pp 161-70.

Bowling, A. (1991) *Measuring health: A review of quality of life measurement scales*, Milton Keynes: Open University Press.

Bowling, A. (1995) *Measuring disease: A review of disease-specific quality of life measurement scales*, Buckingham, PA: Open University Press.

Brage, S., Bjerkedal, T. and Bruusgaard, D. (1997) 'Occupation-specific morbidity of musculoskeletal disease in Norway', *Scandinavian Journal of Social Medicine*, vol 25, pp 50-7.

Braveman, P., Krieger, N. and Lynch, J. (2000) 'Health inequalities and social inequalities in health', *Bulletin of the World Health Organisation*, vol 78, pp 232-4.

Breen, R. and Rottman D. (1995) *Class stratification. A comparative perspective*, London: Harvester Wheatsheaf.

Broadhead, W.E., Kaplan, B.H., Sherman, A.J., Wagner, E.H., Schoenbach, V.J., Grimson, R., Heyden, S., Tibblin, G. and Gehlbach, S.H. (1983) 'The epidemiologic evidence for a relationship between social support and health', *American Journal of Epidemiology*, vol 117, pp 521-37.

Bultmann, U., Kant, I.J., van den Brandt, P.A. and Kasl, S.V. (2002) 'Psychosocial work characteristics as risk factors for the onset of fatigue and psychological distress: prospective results from the Maastricht Cohort Study', *Psychological Medicine*, vol 32, pp 333-45.

Bygren, M. and Duvander, A.-Z. (2004) 'Ingen annan på jobbet har ju varit pappaledig. Papporna, deras arbetsplatser och deras pappaledighetsuttag' ['Nobody else at work has been on paternal leave'], in M. Bygren, M. Gähler and M. Nermo (eds) *Familj och arbete – vardagsliv i förändring. [Family and work – Changes in everyday life]*, Stockholm: SNS Förlag, pp 166-99.

Bygren, M., Gähler, M. and Nermo, M. (2004) 'Familj och arbete – vardagsliv i förändring' [Family and work – Changes in everyday life'], in M. Bygren, M. Gähler and Nermo (eds) *Familj och arbete – vardagsliv i förändring. [Family and work – Changes in everyday life]*, Stockholm: SNS Förlag, pp 11-55.

Cassel, J. (1976) 'The contribution of the social environment to host resistance', *American Journal of Epidemiology*, vol 104, pp 107-23.

Cavelaars, A., Kunst, A., Geurts, J., Helmert, U., Lahelma, E., Lundberg, O., Matheson, J. et al (1998) 'Differences in self-reported morbidity by income level in six European countries', in A. Cavelaars, 'Cross-national comparisons of socio-economic differences in health indicators', Doctoral thesis, Rotterdam: Department of Public Health, Erasmus University Rotterdam.

Chen, C.S. and Stevenson, H.W. (1989) 'Homework: a cross-cultural examination', *Child Development*, vol 60, pp 551-61.

Chumbler, N.R., Rittman, M., van Puymbroeck, M., Vogel, W.B. and Qin, H. (2004) 'The sense of coherence, burden, and depressive symptoms in informal caregivers during the first month after stroke', *International Journal of Geriatric Psychiatry*, vol 19, pp 944-53.

Clayton, D. and Hills, M. (1993) *Statistical models in epidemiology*, Oxford: Oxford University Press.

CO: Children's Ombudsman [Barnombudsmannen] (2004:03) *Barn och unga berättar om stress. Resultat från Barnombudsmannens undersökning bland kontaktklasserna [Children and young people talk about stress. Results from the Children's Ombudsman's research in the contact classes]*, Spring 2003 (www.bo.se).

CO: Children's Ombudsman [Barnombudsmannen] (2004:06) *Upp till 18 – fakta om barn och ungdom [Up to 18 – facts about children and young people]*, Stockholm: Central Statistics.

Cohen, S. and Syme, S.L. (eds) (1985) *Social support and health*, New York, NY: Academic Press.

Cohen, S., Underwood, L.G. and Gottlieb, B.H. (2000) *Social support measurement and intervention*, New York, NY: Oxford University Press.

Coleman, J. (1988) 'Social capital in the creation of human capital', *American Journal of Sociology*, vol 94, supplement, pp 95-120.

Coleman, J.S. (1990) *Foundations of social theory*, Cambridge, MA: Belknap.

Cox, T., Griffiths, A. and Randall, R. (2003) 'A risk management approach to the prevention of work stress', in M. Schabracq, J.A.M. Winnubst and C.L. Cooper (eds) *The handbook of work and health psychology*, Chichester: John Wiley & Sons, pp 191-206.

Cox, T., Griffiths, A. and Rial-González, E. (2000) *Research on work-related stress*, Luxembourg: European Agency for Safety and Health at Work.

Crimmins, E.M. and Saito, Y. (2001) 'Trends in healthy life expectancy in the United States, 1970-1990: gender, racial, and educational differences', *Social Science & Medicine*, vol 52, pp 1629-41.

Currie, C., Hurrelman, K., Settertobulte, W., Smith, R. and Todd, J. (2000) 'Health and health behaviour among young people. Health behaviour in school-aged children: a WHO cross-national study (HBSC)', in C. Currie, K. Hurrelman, W. Settertobulte, R. Smith and J. Todd (eds) *Health policy for children and adolescents issue 1*, WHO policy series, international report.

Dahl, E. and Birkelund, G.E. (1997) 'Health inequalities in later life in a social democratic welfare state', *Social Science and Medicine*, vol 44, pp 871-81.

Dahl, E., Fritzell, J., Lahelma, E., Martikainen, P., Kunst, A. and Mackenbach, J. (2006) 'Welfare state regimes and health inequalities', in J. Siegrist and M. Marmot (eds) *Social inequalities in health: New evidence and policy implications*, Oxford: Oxford University Press.

Dahlberg, R., Karlqvist, L., Bildt, C. and Nykvist, K. (2004) 'Do work technique and musculoskeletal symptoms differ between men and women performing the same type of work tasks?', *Applied Ergonomics*, vol 35, pp 521-9.

Danielson, M. (2003) *Svenska skolbarns hälsovanor 2001/02. Grundrapport* [*Health habits of Swedish schoolchildren. Basic report*], Report 2003:50, Stockholm: National Institute of Public Health.

Danielson, M. and Marklund, U. (2000) *Svenska skolbarns hälsovanor 1997/98* [*Swedish schoolchildren's health habits 1997/98*], Tabellrapport, Stockholm: Folkhälsoinstitutet.

Davey Smith, G. (ed) (2003) *Health inequalities: Lifecourse approaches*, Bristol: The Policy Press.

Davey Smith, G. and Ebrahim, S. (2003) '"Mendelian randomisation": can genetic epidemiology contribute to understanding environmental determinants of disease?', *International Journal of Epidemiology*, vol 32, pp 1-22.

Davey Smith, G., Hart, C., Blane, D., Gillis C. and Hawthorne, V. (1997) 'Lifetime socioeconomic position and mortality: prospective observational study', *British Medical Journal*, vol 314, pp 547-52.

de Jonge, J., Bosma, H., Peter, R. and Siegrist, J. (2000a) 'Job strain, effort-reward imbalance and employee well-being: a large-scale cross-sectional study', *Social Science & Medicine*, vol 50, pp 1317-27.

de Jonge, J., Reuvers, M.M., Houtman, I.L., Bongers, P.M. and Kompier, M.A. (2000b) 'Linear and nonlinear relations between psychosocial job characteristics, subjective outcomes, and sickness absence: baseline results from SMASH', *Journal of Occupational Health Psychology*, vol 5, pp 256–68.

Deaton, A. (2001) 'Relative deprivation, inequality, and mortality', Princeton, Centre for Health and Wellbeing, Working Paper (www.wws.princeton.edu/~chw/research/papers.html).

Deaton A. (2003) 'Health, inequality, and economic development', *Journal of Economic Literature*, vol XLI, pp 113-58.

Denton, M. and Walters, V. (1999) 'Gender differences in structural and behavioral determinants of health: an analysis of the social production of health', *Social Science & Medicine*, vol 48, pp 1221-35.

Denton, M., Prus, S. and Walters, V. (2004) 'Gender differences in health: a Canadian study of the psychosocial, structural and behavioural determinants of health', *Social Science & Medicine*, vol 58, pp 2585-600.

Diderichsen, F. and Dahlgren, G. (1991) 'Klass och ohälsa i ett generationsperspektiv' ['Class and ill health from a generational perspective'], in F. Diderichsen, P. Östlin, G. Dahlgren and C. Hogstedt (eds) *Klass och ohälsa* [*Class and ill health*], Stockholm: Tiden-Folksam, pp 185-206.

Dryler, H. (1998) *Educational choice in Sweden: Studies on the importance of gender and social contexts*, Dissertation Series No 31, Stockholm: Swedish Institute for Social Research.

Due, P., Lynch, J., Holstein, B. and Modvig, J. (2003) 'Socioeconomic health inequalities among a nationally representative sample of Danish adolescents: the role of different types of social relations', *Journal of Epidemiology and Community Health*, vol 57, pp 692-8.

Due, P., Holstein, B., Lund, R., Modvig, J. and Avlund, K. (1999) 'Social relations: network, support and relational strain', *Social Science & Medicine*, vol 48, pp 661-73.

Durkheim, E. (1897/1997) *Suicide: A study in sociology*, New York, NY: Free Press.

Easterlin, R.A. (1980) *Birth and fortune: The impact of numbers on personal welfare*, New York, NY: Basic Books.

Ecob, R. and Davey Smith, G. (1999) 'Income and health: what is the nature of the relationship?', *Social Science & Medicine*, vol 48, pp 693-705.

Edin, P.-A. and Åslund, O. (2001) 'Invandrare på 1990-talets arbetsmarknad' ('Immigrants in the labour market of the 1990s'), in Å. Bergmark (ed) *Ofärd i välfärden* [*Disadvantage in the welfare society*], (SOU) 2001:54, Stockholm: Fritzes.

Eibner, C.E. and Evans, W.N. (2001) 'Relative deprivation, poor health habits and mortality', Princeton, Centre for Health and Wellbeing, Working Paper (www.wws.princeton.edu/~chw/research/papers.html).

Ekberg, K., Bjorkqvist, B., Malm, P., Bjerre-Kiely, B., Karlsson, M. and Axelson, O. (1994) 'Case-control study of risk factors for disease in the neck and shoulder area', *Occupational and Environmental Medicine*, vol 51, pp 262-6.

Elder, G.H. (1974) *Children of the Great Depression*, Chicago, IL: University of Chicago Press.

Elder, G.H. (1995) 'The life course paradigm: social change and individual development', in P. Moen, G.H. Elder and K. Lüscher, *Examining lives in context: Perspectives on the ecology of human development*, Washington, DC: American Psychological Association, pp 101-39.

Ellaway, A., McKay, L., Macintyre, S., Kearns, A. and Hiscock, R. (2004) 'Are social comparisons of homes and cars related to psychosocial health?', *International Journal of Epidemiology*, vol 33, pp 1065-71.

Elstad, J.I. (2001) 'Health-related mobility, health inequalities and gradient constraint', *European Journal of Public Health*, vol 11, pp 135-40.

Elstad, J.I. (2004) 'Health and status attainment: effects of health on occupational achievement among employed Norwegian men', *Acta Sociologica*, vol 47, pp 127-40.

Emslie, C., Hunt, K. and Macintyre, S. (1999) 'Problematizing gender, work and health: the relationship between gender, occupational grade, working conditions and minor morbidity in full-time bank employees', *Social Science & Medicine*, vol 48, pp 33-48.

Emslie, C., Fuhrer, R., Hunt, K., Macintyre, S., Shipley, M. and Stansfeld, S. (2002) 'Gender differences in mental health: evidence from three organisations', *Social Science & Medicine*, vol 54, pp 621-4.

Engels, F. (1969/1845) *The conditions of the working class in England*, London: Panther Books.

Erikson, R. (1984) 'Social class of men, women and families', *Sociology*, vol 18, pp 500-14.

Erikson, R. (2006) 'Social class assignment and mortality in Sweden', *Social Science & Medicine*, vol 62, pp 2151-60.

Erikson, R. and Åberg, R (eds) (1987) *Welfare in transition*, Oxford: Clarendon Press.

Erikson, R. and Goldthorpe, J.H. (1992) *The constant flux. A study of class mobility in industrial societies*, Oxford: Clarendon Press.

Erikson, R. and Tåhlin, M. (1987) 'Coexistence of welfare problems', in R. Erikson and R. Åberg (eds) *Welfare in transition*, Oxford: Clarendon Press.

Erikson, R. and Uusitalo, H. (1987) 'The Scandinavian approach to welfare research', in R. Erikson, E.J. Hansen, S. Ringen and H. Uusitalo (eds) *The Scandinavian model: Welfare states and welfare research*, Armonk: M.E. Sharpe, pp 177-93.

Esping-Andersen, G. (1990) *The three worlds of welfare capitalism*, Oxford: Polity Press.

Esping-Andersen, G. (1999) *Social foundations of postindustrial economies*, Oxford: Oxford University Press.

Esping-Andersen, G. (2000) *Social indicators and welfare monitoring*, Social Policy and Development Programme Paper Number 2, Geneva: UNRISD.

Evertsson, M. (2004) *Facets of gender: Analyses of the family and the labour market*, Stockholm: Swedish Institute for Social Research.

Feldt, T. (1997) 'The role of sense of coherence in well-being at work: analyses of main and moderator effects', *Work and Stress*, vol 11, pp 134-47.

Feldt, T. (2000) *Sense of coherence. Structure, stability, and health promoting role in working life*, Jyväskylä: Department of Psychology, University of Jyväskylä.

Feldt, T., Kinnunen, U. and Mauno, S. (2000a) 'A mediational model of sense of coherence in the work context: a one-year follow-up study', *Journal of Organizational Behavior*, vol 21, pp 461-76.

Feldt, T., Leskinen, E., Kinnunen, U. and Mauno, S. (2000b) 'Longitudinal factor analysis models in the assessment of the stability of sense of coherence', *Personality and Individual Differences*, vol 28, pp 239-57.

Ferrarini, T. (2003) *Parental leave institutions in eighteen post-war welfare states*, Stockholm: Swedish Institute for Social Research.

Feveile, H., Jensen, C. and Burr, H. (2002) 'Risk factors for neck-shoulder and wrist-hand symptoms in a 5-year follow-up study of 3,990 employees in Denmark', *International Archives of Occupational and Environmental Health*, vol 75, pp 243-51.

Finance and Development (2004) 'Freedom as progress, Laura Wallace interviews Nobel Prize-winner Amartya Sen', September, pp 4-7.

Fox, J. (ed) (1989) *Health inequalities in European countries*, Gower: Aldershot.

Fratiglioni, L., Viitanen, M., von Strauss, E., Tontodonati, V., Herlitz, A. and Winblad, B. (1997) 'Very old women at highest risk of dementia and Alzheimer's disease: incidence data from the Kungsholmen Project, Stockholm', *Neurology*, vol 48, pp 132-8.

Freedman, V.A., Crimmins, E., Schoeni, R.F., Spillman, B.C., Aykan, H., Kramarow, E. et al (2004) 'Resolving inconsistencies in trends in old-age disability: report from a technical working group', *Demography*, vol 41, pp 417-41.

Fritzell, J. (2001) 'Inkomstfördelningens trender under 1990-talet' ['Income distribution trends in the 1990s'], in J. Fritzell and J Palme (eds) *Välfärdens finansiering och fördelning* [*The financing and distribution of welfare*], (SOU) 2001:57, Stockholm: Fritzes.

Fritzell, J. and Lennartsson, C. (2005) 'Financial transfers between generations in Sweden', *Ageing and Society*, vol 25, pp 397-414.

Fritzell, J. and Lundberg, O. (1993) *Ett förlorat eller förlovat årtionde? Välfärdsutvecklingen mellan 1981 och 1991* [*A promised or lost decade?*], Stockholm: Swedish Institute for Social Research.

Fritzell, J. and Lundberg, O. (eds) (1994) *Vardagens villkor. Levnadsförhållanden i Sverige undre tre decennier* [*Everyday life. Living conditions in Sweden during three decades*], Stockholm: Brombergs.

Fritzell, J. and Lundberg, O. (2000a) 'The Swedish Level of Living Survey: longitudinal research on life chances over the life course', in C.-G. Janson (ed) *Seven Swedish longitudinal studies in the behavioral sciences*, Stockholm: FRN.

Fritzell, J. and Lundberg, O. (2000b) *Välfärd, ofärd och ojämlikhet* [*Welfare, disadvantage and inequality*], (SOU) 2000:41, Stockholm: Fritzes.

Fritzell, J. and Lundberg, O. (2005) 'Fighting inequalities in health and income – one important road to welfare and social development', in O. Kangas and J. Palme (eds) *Social policy and economic development in the Nordic countries*, Basingstoke: Palgrave, pp 164-85.

Fritzell, J. and Ritakallio, V.-M. (2004) *Societal shifts and changed patterns of poverty*, LIS Working Paper 393, Syracuse, NY: Syracuse University.

Fritzell, J., Nermo, M. and Lundberg, O. (2004) 'The impact of income: assessing the relationship between income and health in Sweden', *Scandinavian Journal of Public Health*, vol 32, pp 6-16.

Fuhrer, R. and Stansfeld, S.A. (2002) 'How gender affects patterns of social relations and their impact on health: a comparison of one or multiple sources of support from "close persons"', *Social Science & Medicine*, vol 54, pp 811-25.

Fuhrer, R., Stansfeld, S.A., Chemali, J. and Shipley, M.J. (1999) 'Gender, social relations and mental health: prospective findings from an occupational cohort (Whitehall II study)', *Social Science & Medicine*, vol 48, pp 77-87.

Fukuyama, F. (1995) *Trust – The social virtues and the creation of prosperity*, London: Penguin Books.

Fukuyama, F. (2000) *Social capital and civil society*, IMF Working Paper No 00/74, Washington, DC: IMF [unpublished].

Galobardes, B., Lynch, J.W. and Davey Smith, G. (2004) 'Childhood socioeconomic circumstances and cause-specific mortality in adulthood: systematic review and interpretation', *Epidemiological Reviews*, vol 26, pp 7-21.

Gerdtham, U.G. and Johannesson, M. (2004) 'Absolute income, relative income, income inequality and mortality', *Journal of Human Resources*, vol 39, pp 228-47.

Gilbar, O. (1998) 'Relationship between burnout and sense of coherence in health social workers', *Social Work in Health Care*, vol 26, pp 39-49.

Gillander Gådin, K. (2002) 'Does the psychosocial school environment matter for health? A study of pupils in Swedish contemporary school from a gender perspective', Doctoral dissertation, Umeå University.

Gillander Gådin, K. and Hammarström, A. (2000) 'School-related health – a cross-sectional study among young boys and girls', *International Journal of Health Services*, vol 30, pp 797-820.

Gillander Gådin, K. and Hammarström, A. (2003) 'Do changes in the psychosocial school environment influence pupils' health development? Results from a three-year follow-up study', *Scandinavian Journal of Public Health*, vol 31, pp 169-77.

Goldman, N., Korenman, S. and Weinstein, R. (1995) 'Marital status and health among the elderly', *Social Science & Medicine*, vol 40, pp 1717-30.

Goodman, E., Huang, B., Wade, T.J. and Kahn, R.S. (2003) 'A multilevel analysis of the relation of socioeconomic status to adolescent depressive symptoms: does school context matter?', *Journal of Paediatrics*, vol 143, pp 451-6.

Gore, S., Aseltine, R.H. and Colten, M.E. (1992) 'Social structure, life stress, and depressive symptoms in a high school-age population', *Journal of Health and Social Behavior*, vol 33, pp 97-113.

Gornick, J.C. and Meyers, M.K. (2003) *Families that work: Policies for reconciling parenthood and employment*, New York, NY: Russell Sage.

Granovetter, M. (1973) 'The strength of weak ties', *American Journal of Sociology*, vol 78, pp 1360-80.

Grundy, E. and Sloggett, A. (2003) 'Health inequalities in the older population: the role of personal capital, social resources and socio-economic circumstances', *Social Science & Medicine*, vol 56, pp 935-47.

Grusky, D (2001) 'The past, present and future of social inequality', in D. Grusky (ed) *Social stratification in sociological perspective*, Boulder, CO: Westview Press.

Häkkänen, M., Viikari-Juntura, E. and Martikainen, R. (2001) 'Incidence of musculoskeletal disorders among newly employed manufacturing workers', *Scandinavian Journal of Work, Environment and Health*, vol 27, pp 381-7.

Hall, E.M. (1992) 'Double exposure: the combined impact of the home and work environments on psychosomatic strain in Swedish women and men', *International Journal of Health Services*, vol 22, pp 239-60.

Halleröd, B. (1998) 'Poor Swedes, poor Britons: a comparative analysis of relative deprivation', in H. Andreβ (ed) *Empirical poverty research in a comparative perspective*, Aldershot: Ashgate.

Halleröd, B., Marklund, S., Nordlund, A. and Stattin, M. (1993) *Konsensuell fattigdom – en studie av konsumtion och attityder till konsumtion. [Consensual poverty – a study of consumption and attitudes towards consumption]*. Umeå Studies in Sociology, 1993:104. Umeå: Umeå University.

Hallqvist, J., Lynch, J., Bartley, M., Lang, T. and Blane, D. (2003) 'Accumulation of exposure to low socioeconomic positions during the life course and risk of myocardial infarction. Can the effect be disentangled from effects of critical periods and social mobility?', *Social Science & Medicine*, vol 58, pp 1555-62.

Hansell, S. (1985) 'Adolescent friendship networks and distress in school', *Social Forces*, vol 63, pp 698-715.

Harpham, T., Grant, E. and Thomas, E. (2002) 'Measuring social capital within health surveys: key issues', *Health Policy Plan*, vol 17, pp 106-11.

Haugland, S., Wold, B., Stevenson, J., Aaroe, L.E. and Woynarowska, B. (2001) 'Subjective health complaints in adolescence', *European Journal of Public Health*, vol 11, pp 4-10.

Hemmingsson, T. and Lundberg, I. (2005) 'How far are socioeconomic differences in coronary heart disease hospitalization, all-cause mortality and cardiovascular mortality among adult Swedish males attributable to negative childhood circumstances and behaviour in adolescence?', *International Journal of Epidemiology*, vol 34, pp 260-7.

Hemström, Ö. (1998) *Male susceptibility and female emancipation*, Stockholm: Almqvist & Wiksell International.

Hemström, Ö. (1999) 'Does the work environment contribute to excess male mortality?', *Social Science & Medicine*, vol 49, pp 879-94.

Hemström, Ö. (2001a) 'Class differences in morbidity and mortality', in S. Marklund (ed) *Worklife and health in Sweden 2000*, Stockholm: National Institute for Working Life, pp 135-54.

Hemström, Ö. (2001b) 'Working conditions, the work environment and health', *Scandinavian Journal of Public Health*, vol 29, Supplement 58, pp 167-84.

Hemström, Ö. (2002) 'Långtidssjukskrivna, förtidspensionärer, långtidsarbetslösa och långtidsfriska' [An analysis of individuals on long-term sickness absence, early retirement, long-term unemployment and the long-term healthy], in *Handlingsplan för ökad hälsa i arbetslivet [Action programme for improved health in working life]*, (SOU) 2002:5, Del 2, Bilagor, Stockholm: Fritzes Offentliga Publikationer, pp 169-238.

Hemström, Ö. (2005) 'Health inequalities and income in Sweden: the role of work environment', *Social Science and Medicine*, vol 61, pp 637-47.

Hernes, H.M. (1987) *Welfare state and women power*, Oslo: Norwegian University Press.

Hibbard, J.H. and Pope, C.R. (1983) 'Gender roles, illness orientation and use of medical services', *Social Science & Medicine*, vol 17, pp 129-37.

Hinrichs, K. and Kangas, O. (2003) 'When is a change big enough to be a system shift? Small system-shifting changes in German and Finnish pension policies', Social Policy & Administration, vol 37, pp 573-91.

Hoge, T. and Bussing, A. (2004) 'The impact of sense of coherence and negative affectivity on the work stressor—strain relationship', *Journal of Occupational Health Psychology*, vol 9, pp 195-205.

Holmberg, S. and Weibull, L. (2001) 'Land, du välsignade?' ['Thou blessed country?'], in S. Holmberg and L. Weibull (eds) *Land, Du välsignade [Thou blessed country?]*, SOM-report No 26, Göteborg: SOM-institutet.

Holmstrom, E.B., Lindell, J. and Moritz, U. (1992) 'Low back and neck/shoulder pain in construction workers: occupational workload and psychosocial risk factors. Part 1: Relationship to low back pain', *Spine*, vol 17, pp 663-71.

Hoogendoorn, W.E., Bongers, P.M., de Vet, H.C., Douwes, M., Koes, B.W., Miedema, M.C., Ariens, G.A. and Bouter, L.M. (2000) 'Flexion and rotation of the trunk and lifting at work are risk factors for low back pain: results of a prospective cohort study', *Spine*, vol 25, pp 3087-92.

Hörnqvist, M. (1994) 'Att bli vuxen i olika generationer' ['To become adult in different generations'], in J. Fritzell and O. Lundberg, (eds) *Vardagens villkor. Levnadsförhållanden i Sverige undre tre decennier [Everyday life. Living conditions in Sweden during three decades]*, Stockholm: Brombergs, pp 184-214.

Hosmer, D.W. and Lemeshow, S. (1992) 'Confidence interval estimation of interaction', *Epidemiology*, vol 3, pp 452-6.

House, J.S., Kessler, R.C. and Herzog, A.R. (1990) 'Age, socioeconomic status, and health', *Milbank Quarterly*, vol 68, pp 383-411.

House, J.S., Landis, K.R. and Umberson, D. (1988) 'Social relationships and health', *Science,* vol 214, pp 540-5.

Hraba, J., Lorenz, F., Lee, G. and Pechaèová, Z. (1996) 'Gender differences in health: evidence from the Czech Republic', *Social Science & Medicine*, vol 43, pp 1443-51.

Huisman, M., Kunst, A.E. and Mackenbach, J.P. (2003) 'Socioeconomic inequalities in morbidity among the elderly: a European overview', *Social Science and Medicine*, vol 57, pp 861-73.

Huisman, M., Kunst, A.E., Andersen, O., Bopp, M., Borgan, J.K., Borrell, C., Costa, G. et al (2004) 'Socioeconomic inequalities in mortality among elderly people in 11 European populations', *Journal of Epidemiology and Community Health*, vol 58, pp 468-75.

Huisman, M., Kunst, A.E., Bopp, M., Borgan, J.K., Borrell, C., Costa, G. et al (2005) 'Educational inequalities in cause-specific mortality in middle-aged and older men and women in eight western European populations', *Lancet*, vol 365, pp 493-500.

Hyppä, M.T. and Mäki, J. (2001) 'Individual-level relationships between social capital and self rated health in a bilingual community', *Preventive Medicine*, vol 32, pp 148-55.

Illsley, R (1955) 'Social class selection and class differences in relation to stillbirths and infant deaths', *British Medical Journal*, vol 2, pp 1520-4.

Inghe, G. and Inghe, M.-B. (1967) *Den ofärdiga välfärden* [*The unfinished welfare*], Stockholm: Tidens Förlag Folksam.

Jansson, K. (2000) 'Inkomstfördelning under 1990-talet' ['Distribution of income in the 1990s]', in Å. Bergmark (ed) *Välfärd och försörjning* [*Welfare, income and income maintenance*], (SOU) 2000:40, Stockholm: Fritzes.

Job Stress Network (2005) www.workhealth.org, Santa Monica: Center for Social Epidemiology, updated 26 August 2005, accessed 29 August 2005.

Johansson, S. (1970) *Om levnadsnivåundersökningen* [*On the Level-of-Living Survey*], Stockholm: Allmänna förlaget.

Johnson, J.V. (1986) 'The impact of workplace social support, job demands and work control upon cardiovascular disease in Sweden', Doctoral dissertation, Organizational and Environmental Psychology Research Reports No 1, Stockholm, Department of Psychology, Stockholm University.

Jonsson, J.O. and Mills, C. (eds) (2001) *Cradle to grave*, York: Sociology Press.

Jonsson, J.O. and Östberg, V. with M. Evertsson and S. Brolin Låftman, (2001) *Barns och ungdomars välfärd* [*The welfare of children and young people*], (SOU) 2001:55, Stockholm: Fritzes.

Kalimo, R. and Vuori, J. (1990) 'Work and sense of coherence: resources for competence and life satisfaction', *Behavioral Medicine*, vol 16, pp 76-89.

Kalimo, R., Pahkin, K. and Mutanen, P. (2002) 'Work and personal resources as long-term predictors of well-being', *Stress and Health*, vol 18, pp 227-34.

Kalimo, R., Pahkin, K., Mutanen, P. and Torppinen-Tanner, S. (2003) 'Staying well or burning out at work: work characteristics and personal resources as long-term predictors', *Work & Stress*, vol 17, pp 109-22.

Kangas, O. and Palme, J. (2000) 'Does social policy matter? Poverty cycles in the OECD countries', *International Journal of Health Services*, vol 30, pp 335-52.

Kangas, O. and Palme, J. (2005) 'Coming late – catching up: the formation of a "Nordic model"', in O. Kangas and J. Palme (eds) *Social policy and economic development in the Nordic countries*, Basingstoke: Palgrave, pp 17-59.

Karasek, R. (1979) 'Job demands, job decision latitude, and mental strain: implications for job redesign', *Administrative Science Quarterly*, vol 24, pp 285-310.

Karasek, R.A. and Theorell, T. (1990) *Healthy work: Stress, productivity and reconstruction of working life*, New York, NY: Basic Books.

Karasek, R.A. and Theorell, T. (2000) 'The demand-control-support model and CVD', in P. Schnall, K. Belkic, P. Landsbergis, and D. Baker (eds) *The workplace and cardiovascular disease. Occupational medicine (state of the art reviews), 15:1*, Philadelphia, PA: Hanley & Belfus, Inc, pp 78-83.

Karasek, R.A., Theorell, T.G., Schwartz, J., Pieper, C. and Alfredsson, L. (1982) 'Job, psychological factors and coronary heart disease. Swedish prospective findings and US prevalence findings using a new occupational inference method', *Adv Cardiol*, vol 29, pp 62-7.

Kåreholt, I. (2000) *Social class and mortality risk*, Dissertation Series, No 44, Stockholm: Swedish Institute for Social Research.

Kåreholt, I. (2001) 'The long shadow of socioeconomic conditions in childhood: do they affect class inequalities in mortality?', in J.O. Jonsson and C. Mills (eds) *Cradle to grave*, York: Sociology Press.

Karvonen, S., Vikat, A. and Rimpelä, M. (2005) 'The role of school context in the increase in young people's health complaints in Finland', *Journal of Adolescence*, vol 28, pp 1-16.

Kautto, M., Fritzell, J., Hvinden, B., Kvist, J. and Uusitalo, H. (eds) (2001) *Nordic welfare sates in the European context*, London: Routledge.

Kautto, M., Heikkilä, M., Hvinden, B., Marklund, S. and Ploug, N. (eds) (1999) *Nordic social policy: Changing welfare states*, London: Routledge.

Kawachi, I. (2000) 'Income inequality and health', in L.F. Berkman and I. Kawachi (eds) *Social epidemiology*, New York, NY: Oxford University Press.

Kawachi, I. and Berkman, L. (2000) 'Social cohesion, social capital, and health', in L. Berkman and I. Kawachi (eds) *Social epidemiology*, Oxford: Oxford University Press, pp 174-90.

Kawachi, I., Kennedy, B.P. and Glass, R. (1999a) 'Social capital and self-rated health: a contextual analysis', *American Journal of Public Health*, vol 89, pp 1187-93.

Kawachi, I., Kennedy, B.P. and Wilkinson, R.G. (1999b) 'Crime: social disorganisation and relative deprivation', *Social Science & Medicine*, vol 48, pp 719-31.

Kawachi, I., Subramanian, S.V. and Almeida-Filho, N. (2002) 'A glossary for health inequalities', *Journal of Epidemiology and Community Health*, vol 56, pp 647-52.

Kennely, B., O'Shea, E. and Garvey, E. (2003) 'Social capital, life expectancy and mortality: a cross-national examination', *Social Science & Medicine*, vol 56, pp 2367-77.

Kenworthy, L. (2004) *Egalitarian capitalism*, New York, NY: Russell Sage.

Kildal, N. and Kuhnle, S (eds) (2005) *Normative foundations of the welfare state: The Nordic experience*, London: Routledge.

Kivimäki, M., Feldt, T., Vahtera, J. and Nurmi, J.-E. (2000) 'Sense of coherence and health: evidence from two cross-lagged longitudinal samples', *Social Science & Medicine*, vol 50, pp 583-97.

Kjeldstad, R. (2001) 'Gender policies and gender equality', in M. Kautto, J. Fritzell, B. Hvinden, J. Kvist and H. Uusitalo (eds) *Nordic welfare states in the European context*, London: Routledge.

Klausen, K.K. and Selle, P. (1995) *Frivillig organisering i norden* [*Voluntary organisation in the Nordic countries*], Köpenhamn: Jurist och ekonomförbundets Förlag.

Kohli, M. (1999) 'Private and public transfers between generations: linking the family and the state', *European Societies*, vol 1, pp 81-104.

Korpi, W. (2000) 'Faces of inequality: gender, class and patterns of inequalities in different type of welfare state', *Social Politics*, vol 7, pp 127-91.

Korpi, W. and Palme, J. (1998) 'The paradox of redistribution and strategies of equality: welfare state institutions, inequality and poverty in the western countries', *American Sociological Review*, vol 63, pp 661-87.

Krantz, G. and Östergren, P.-O. (1999) 'Women's health: do common symptoms in women mirror general distress or specific disease entities?', *Scandinavian Journal of Public Health*, vol 27, pp 311-17.

Krantz, G., Berntsson, L. and Lundberg, U. (2005) 'Total workload, work stress and perceived symptoms in Swedish male and female white-collar employees', *European Journal of Public Health*, vol 15, pp 209-14.

Krieger, N. (2003) 'Genders, sexes, and health: what are the connections – and why does it matter?', *International Journal of Epidemiology*, vol 32, pp 652-7.

Kristensen, T., Bjorner, J.B., Christensen, K.B. and Borg, W. (2004) 'The distinction between work pace and working hours in the measurement of quantitative demands at work', *Work & Stress*, vol 18, pp 305-22.

Kuh, D., Ben-Shlomo, Y., Lynch, J., Hallqvist, J. and Power, C. (2003) 'Life course epidemiology', *Journal of Epidemiology and Community Health*, vol 57, pp 778-83.

Kuhn, T. (1970) *The structure of scientific revolutions*, Chicago, IL: University of Chicago Press.

Kuhnle, S. (ed) (2000) *Survival of the European welfare state*, London: Routledge.

Kuhnle, S. and Alestalo, M. (2000) 'Introduction: growth, adjustments and survival of European welfare states', in S. Kuhnle (ed) *Survival of the European welfare state*, London: Routledge, pp 3-18.

Kunst A., Groenhof, F., Mackenbach, J. and the EU Working Group on Socioeconomic Inequalities in Health (1998) 'Mortality by occupational class among men 30-64 years in 11 European countries', *Social Science & Medicine*, vol 46, pp 1459-76.

Låftman, Brolin S. (2005) 'Effort and reward in school. The psychosocial work environment and health of 10-18 year old girls and boys' (unpublished).

Låftman, Brolin S. and Östberg, V. (2006) 'The pros and cons of social relations. An analysis of adolescents' health complaints', *Social Science and Medicine,* vol 63, pp 611-23.

Lahelma, E. (2001) 'Health and social stratification', in W. Cockerham (ed) *The Blackwell companion to medical sociology*, Oxford: Blackwell.

Lahelma, E., Martikainen, P., Rahkonen, O. and Silventoinen, K. (1999) 'Gender differences in ill health in Finland: patterns, magnitude and change', *Social Science & Medicine*, vol 48, pp 7-19.

Lahelma, E., Arber, S., Martikainen, P., Rahkonen, O. and Silventoinen, K. (2001) 'The myth of gender differences in health: social structural determinants across adult ages in Britain and Finland', *Current Sociology*, vol 49, pp 31-54.

Laslett, P. (1987) 'The emergence of the third age', *Ageing and Society*, vol 7, pp 133-60.

le Grand, C. (1991) 'Explaining the male-female wage gap: job segregation and solidarity wage bargaining in Sweden', *Acta Sociologica*, vol 34, pp 261-78.

le Grand, C., Szulkin, R. and Tåhlin, M. (2001) 'Har jobben blivit bättre? En analys av arbetsinnehållet under tre decennier' ['Have the jobs become better? An analysis of work content during three decades'], in J. Fritzell, M. Gähler, and O. Lundberg (eds) *Välfärd och arbete i arbetslöshetens årtionde: Antologi från Kommittén Välfärdsbokslut* [*Welfare and work in a decade of unemployment*], Reports of the Government Commissions, (SOU) 2001:53, Stockholm: Fritzes, pp 79-117.

le Grand, C., Szulkin, R. and Tåhlin, M. (2004) 'Överutbildning eller kompetensbrist? Matchning på den svenska arbetsmarknaden 1974-2000' ['Over-education or competence shortage? Matching on the Swedish labour market 1974-2000'], in M. Bygren, M. Gähler and M. Nermo (eds) *Familj och arbete – vardagsliv i förändring* [*Family and work – everyday life in transition*], Stockholm: SNS Förlag, pp 283-321.

Levi, L. (1984) *Stress in industry: Causes, effects, and prevention*, Geneva: International Labour Office.

Levi, L. (2002) Personal communication at Seminarium 'Ledarskap-Arbete-Hälsa', [Leadership-Work-Health] Stockholm, 23 May 2002.

Li, Y., Pickles, A. and Savage, M. (2005) 'Social capital and social trust in Britain', *European Sociological Review*, vol 21, pp 109-23.

Lidwall, U. and Skogman Thoursie, P. (2000) 'Sjukskrivningar och förtidspensionering under de senaste decennierna' [Sick leave and early retirement during the last decades'], in S. Marklund (ed) *Arbetsliv och hälsa 2000* [*Work life and health 2000*], Stockholm: Arbetslivsinstitutet, pp 91-124.

Lidwall, U., Marklund, S. and Skogman Thoursie, P. (2004) 'Utvecklingen av sjukfrånvaron i Sverige' ['The development of sickness absence in Sweden'], in R.Å. Gustafsson, and I. Lundberg (eds) *Arbetsliv och hälsa 2004 [Work life and health 2004]*, Stockholm: National Institute for Working Life, pp 173-93.

Lieberson, S. (1985) *Making it count*, Berkeley, CA: University of California Press.

Lin, N. (2000) 'Inequality in Social Capital', *Contemporary Sociology*, vol 29, pp 785-95.

Lin, N. (2001) *Social capital: A theory of structure and action*, Cambridge: Cambridge University Press.

Lindfors, P., Lundberg, O. and Lundberg, U. (2005) 'Sense of coherence and biomarkers of health in 43-year-old women', *International Journal of Behavioral Medicine*, vol 12 pp 98-103.

Lindström, M., Hanson, B.S. and Östergren, P.-O. (2001) 'Socioeconomic differences in leisure-time physical activity: the role of social participation and social capital in shaping health related behaviour', *Social Science & Medicine*, vol 52, pp 441-51.

Lindström, M., Hanson, B.S., Östergren, P.-O. and Berglund, G. (2000) 'Socioeconomic differences in smoking cessation: the role of social participation', *Scandinavian Journal of Public Health*, vol 28, pp 200-8.

Link, B. and Phelan, J. (1995) 'Social conditions as fundamental causes of disease', *Journal of Health and Social Behavior*, vol 35 (extra issue), pp 80-94.

Lipset, S.M. and Bendix, R. (1952) 'Social mobility and occupational career patterns', *American Journal of Sociology*, vol 57, pp 366-74.

Lipset, S.M. and Bendix, R. (1959) *Social mobility in industrial society*, Berkeley and Los Angeles, CA: University of California Press.

Litwin, H. (1998) 'Social network type and health status in a national sample of elderly Israelis', *Social Science & Medicine*, vol 46, pp 599-609.

Ljung, R. and Hallqvist, J. (2006) 'Accumulation of adverse socioeconomic position over the entire life course and the risk of myocardial infarction among men and women', *Journal of Epidemiology and Community Health* (in press).

Lochner, K., Kawachi, I. and Kennedy, B.P. (1999) 'Social capital: a guide to its measurement', *Health and Place*, vol 5, pp 1181-8.

Lopez-Claros, A. and Zahidi, S. (2005) *Women's empowerment: Measuring the global gender gap*, Geneva: World Economic Forum.

Lundberg, M., Fredlund, P., Hallqvist, J. and Diderichsen, F. (1996) 'A SAS program calculating three measures of interaction with confidence intervals', *Epidemiology*, vol 7, pp 655-6.

Lundberg, O. (1986) 'Class and health: comparing Britain and Sweden', *Social Science & Medicine*, vol 26, pp 511-17.

Lundberg, O. (1990) *Den ojämlika ohälsan: om klass- och könsskillnader i sjuklighet [Inequalities in ill health: On class and sex differences in illness]*, Stockholm: Almqvist & Wiksell International.

Lundberg, O. (1991) 'Childhood living conditions, health status and social mobility: a contribution to the health selection debate', *European Sociological Review*, vol 7, pp 149-61.

Lundberg, O. (1993) 'The impact of childhood living conditions on illness and mortality in adulthood', *Social Science & Medicine*, vol 36, pp 1047-52.

Lundberg, O. (1997) 'Childhood conditions, sense of coherence, social class and adult ill health: exploring their theoretical and empirical relations', *Social Science & Medicine*, vol 44, pp 821-31.

Lundberg, O. and Kåreholt, I. (1996) 'The social patterning of mortality in a cohort of elderly Swedes', *Yearbook of Population Research in Finland*, vol 33.

Lundberg, O. and Lahelma, E. (2001) 'Nordic health inequalities in the European context', in M. Kautto, J. Fritzell, B. Hvinden, J. Kvist and H. Uusitalo (eds) *Nordic welfare states in the European context*, London: Routledge.

Lundberg, O. and Nyström Peck, M. (1994) 'Sense of coherence, social structure and health', *European Journal of Public Health*, vol 4, pp 252-7.

Lundberg, O. and Nyström Peck, M. (1995) 'A simplified way of measuring sense of coherence', *European Journal of Public Health*, vol 5, pp 56-9.

Lundberg, O. and Thorslund, M. (1996a) 'Fieldwork and measurement considerations in surveys of the oldest old. Experiences from the Swedish Level of Living Surveys', *Social Indicators Research*, vol 37, pp 165-7.

Lundberg, O. and Thorslund, M. (1996b) 'Inkomst som mått på vårdbehov – kan resurserna för vård av äldre fördelas bättre?' ['Income as a measure of need for care – can resources for care of the elderly be distributed in a better way?'], *Läkartidningen*, vol 93, pp 2606-8.

Lundberg, U. (2002) 'Psychophysiology of work: stress, gender, endocrine response, and work-related upper extremity disorders', *American Journal of Industrial Medicine*, vol 41, pp 383-92.

Lynch, J.W., Davey Smith, G., Kaplan, G.A. and House J.S, (2000) 'Income inequality and mortality: importance to health of individual income, psychosocial environment, or material conditions', *British Medical Journal*, vol 320, pp 1200-4.

Lynch, J., Davey Smith, G., Harper, S., Hillemeier, M., Ross, N., Kaplan, G. and Wolfson, M. (2004) 'Is income inequality a determinant of population health? Part 1. A systematic review', *The Milbank Quarterly*, vol 82, pp 5-99.

McDonough, P. and Walters, V. (2001) 'Gender differences in health: reassessing patterns and explanations', *Social Science & Medicine*, vol 52, pp 547-59.

Macintyre, S. (1992) 'The effects of family position and status on health', *Social Science & Medicine*, vol 35, pp 453-64.

Macintyre, S. (1993) 'Gender differences in the perceptions of common cold symptoms', *Social Science & Medicine*, vol 36, pp 15-20.

Macintyre, S. (1997) 'The Black Report and beyond: what are the issues?', *Social Science & Medicine*, vol 44, pp 723-45.

Macintyre, S., Ford, G. and Hunt, K. (1999) 'Do women "over-report" morbidity? Men's and women's responses to structured prompting on a standard question on longstanding illness', *Social Science & Medicine*, vol 48, pp 89-98.

Macintyre, S., Hunt, K. and Sweeting, H. (1996) 'Gender differences in health: are things really as simple as they seem?', *Social Science & Medicine*, vol 42, pp 617-24.

Mack, J. and Lansley, S. (1985) *Poor Britain*, London: George Allen & Unwin Ltd.

Mackenbach, J.P. (2002) 'Income inequality and population health', *British Medical Journal*, vol 324, pp 1-2.

Mackenbach, J.P. (2005a) *Health inequalities: Europe in profile*, Published under the auspices of the UK Presidency of the EU, London: DH Publications.

Mackenbach, J.P. (2005b) 'Odol, Autobahne and a non-smoking Führer: Reflections on the innocence of public health', *International Journal of Epidemiology*, vol 34, pp 537-9.

Mackenbach, J.P., Kunst, A.E., Cavelaars, A.E.J.M., Groenhof, F. and Geurts, J. (1997) 'Socioeconomic inequalities in morbidity and mortality in western Europe', *Lancet*, vol 7, pp 1655-9.

Malthus, T.R. (1926/1798) *First essay on population*, London: Macmillan.

Marmot, M.G. (2004) *Status syndrome. How your social standing directly affects your health*, London: Bloomsbury.

Marmot, M.G., Kogevinas, M. and Elston, M.A. (1987) 'Social/economic status and disease', *Annual Review of Public Health*, vol 8, pp 111-35.

Marshall, T.H. (1950) *Citizenship and social class and other essays*, Cambridge: Cambridge University Press.

Martikainen, P., Martelin, T., Nihtila, E., Majamaa, K. and Koskinen, S. (2005) 'Differences in mortality by marital status in Finland from 1976 to 2000: analyses of changes in marital-status distributions, socio-demographic and household composition, and cause of death', *Population Studies (Camb)*, vol 59, pp 99-115.

Mayer, K.U. (2001) 'The paradox of global social change and national path dependencies: life course patterns in advanced societies', in A.E. Woodward and M. Kohli (eds) *Inclusions and exclusions in European societies*, London: Routledge, pp 89-110.

MHSA (Ministry of Health and Social Affairs) (2005) 'Policy for the elderly', Fact sheet No 14, Stockholm: Regeringskansliet.

Modin, B. (2003) 'Born out of wedlock and never married – it breaks a man's heart', *Social Science and Medicine*, vol 57, pp 487-501

Moen, P., Elder, G.H. and Lüscher, K. (1995) *Examining lives in context. Perspectives on the ecology of human development*, Washington, DC: American Psychological Association.

Montanari, I. (2000) *Social citizenship and work in welfare states: Comparative studies on convergence and on gender*, Dissertation Series No 45, Stockholm: Swedish Institute for Social Research.

Montanari, I. (2001) 'Choosing time and time for work: cross–national variation in paid work among married women', *Sociologisk forskning*, vol 38, pp 6-31.

Muhonen, T. and Torkelson, E. (2003) 'The demand–control–support model and health among women and men in similar occupations', *Journal of Behavioural Medicine*, vol 26, pp 601-13.

Murphy, M., Glaser, K. and Grundy, E. (1997) 'Marital status and long-term illness in Great Britain', *Journal of Marriage and Family*, vol 59, pp 156-64.

Murray, C., Gakidou, E. and Frenk, J. (1999) 'Health inequalities and social group differences: what should we measure?', *Bulletin of the World Health Organisation*, vol 77, pp 537-43.

Mussweiler, T. (2003) 'Comparison processes in social judgement: mechanisms and consequences', *Psychological Review*, vol 110, pp 472-89.

NAE National Agency for Education [Skolverket] (2001) *Attityder till skolan 2001 [Attitudes towards school 2001]*, Report No 197, Stockholm: Skolverket.

NAE (2003) *Barnomsorg, skola och vuxenutbildning [Childcare, school and adult education]*, Report No 238, Stockholm: Fritzes.

NAE (2004a) *Attityder till skolan 2003 [Attitudes towards school 2003]*, Report No 243, Stockholm: Fritzes.

NAE (2004b) *Slutbetyg från grundskolan våren 2003 [Final grades in elementary school, spring 2003]*, Promemoria of 2 October 2004, Stockholm: Skolverket.

Nakamura, H., Matsuzaki, I., Sasahara, S., Hatta, K., Nagase, H., Oshita, Y., Ogawa, Y., Nobukuni, Y., Kambayashi, Y. and Ogino, K. (2003) 'Enhancement of a sense of coherence and natural killer cell activity which occurred in subjects who improved their exercise habits through health education in the workplace', *Journal of Occupational Health*, vol 45, pp 278-85.

Näringsdepartementet (Ministry of Industry, Employment and Communications) (2000) *Ett föränderligt arbetsliv på gott och ont: utvecklingen av den stressrelaterade ohälsan [A changing working life for better or worse: The development of stress-related ill health]*, Ds 2000:54, Stockholm: Fritzes.

Nasermoaddeli, A., Sekine, M., Hamanishi, S. and Kagamimori, S. (2003) 'Associations between sense of coherence and psychological work characteristics with changes in quality of life in Japanese civil servants: a 1-year follow-up study', *Industrial Health*, vol 41, pp 236-41.

Natvig, G.K., Albrektsen, G., Anderssen, N. and Qvarnstrøm, U. (1999) 'School-related stress and psychosomatic symptoms among school adolescents', *Journal of School Health*, vol 69, pp 362-8.

Nazroo, J.Y., Edwards, A.C. and Brown, G.W. (1998) 'Gender differences in the prevalence of depression: artefact, alternative disorders, biology or roles?', *Sociology of Health & Illness*, vol 20, pp 312-30.

NBHW (2001) *Folkhälsorapport 2001 [Public health report 2001]*, Stockholm: Socialstyrelsen och EpC [National Board of Health and Welfare].

NBHW (2005a) *Folkhälsorapport 2005 [Public health report 2005]*, Stockholm: Socialstyrelsen och EpC [National Board of Health and Welfare].

NBHW (2005b) *Äldre – vård och omsorg år 2004* [*Care and services for elderly people 2004*], Stockholm: Socialstyrelsen och EpC [National Board of Health and Welfare].

NBHW (2006) *Social rapport 2006* [*Social report 2006*], Stockholm: Socialstyrelsen och EpC [National Board of Health and Welfare].

Nermo, M. (1999) *Structured by gender. Patterns of sex segregation in the Swedish labour market. Historical and cross-national comparisons*, Stockholm: Swedish Institute for Social Research.

Niedhammer, I., Landre, M.F., LeClerc, A., Bourgeois, F., Franchi, P., Chastang, J.F., Marignac, G., Mereau, P., Quinton, D., Du Noyer, C.R., Schmaus, A. and Vallayer, C. (1998) 'Shoulder disorders related to work organization and other occupational factors among supermarket cashiers', *International Journal of Occupational and Environmental Health*, vol 4, pp 168-78.

Nilsson, I., Axelsson, K., Gustafson, Y., Lundman, B. and Norberg, A. (2001) 'Well-being, sense of coherence, and burnout in stroke victims and spouses during the first few months after stroke', *Scandinavian Journal of Caring Sciences*, vol 15, pp 203-14.

Nolan, B. and Whelan, C. (1996) *Resources, deprivation and poverty*, Oxford: Clarendon Press.

OECD (Organisation for Economic Co-operation and Development) (2005) *Trends in international migration: SOPEMI*, Paris: OECD.

Olsen, O. (1993) 'Impact of social network on cardiovascular mortality in middle-aged Danish men', *Journal of Epidemiological and Community Health*, vol 47, pp 176-80.

Orloff, A.S. (1993) 'Gender and the social rights of citizenship: the comparative analysis of gender relations and welfare states', *American Sociological Review*, vol 58, pp 303-28.

Östberg, V. (2001a) 'Hälsa och välbefinnande' ['Health and wellbeing'], in *Barns och ungdomars välfärd,* (SOU) 2001:55, Stockholm: Fritzes, pp 239-63.

Östberg, V. (2001b) *Vardagen i skolan: arbetsmiljö, vänner och mobbning* [*Everyday life in school: work environment, friends and bullying*], in (SOU) 2001:55, Kommittén Välfärdsbokslut, Stockholm: Fritzes.

Östberg, V. (2003) 'Children in classrooms: peer status, status distribution and mental well-being', *Social Science & Medicine*, vol 56, pp 17-29.

Östberg, V., Alfvén, G. and Hjern, A. (2006) 'Living conditions and psychosomatic complaints in Swedish school children', *Acta Paediatrica*, vol 95, pp 929-34.

Ouvinen-Birgerstam, P. (1985) *Jag tycker jag är* [*I think I am*], Stockholm: Psykologiförlaget AB.

Pagano, M. and Gauvreau, K. (2000) *Principles of biostatistics*, Pacific Grove, CA: Duxbury.

Palme, J. (2003) 'Pension reform in Sweden and the changing boundaries between public and private', in G.L. Clark and N. Whiteside (eds) *Pension security in the 21st century*, Oxford: Oxford University Press, pp 144-67.

Palme, J., Lundberg, O., Vågerö, D. and Hemström, Ö. (1997) *Klasskillnaderna i ohälsa och dödlighet kräver robust finansiering av förtidspensionerna* [*Class inequalities in health and mortality calls for robust financing of early retirement pensions*], in (SOU) 1997:166, Stockholm: Fritzes, pp 603-22.

Palme, J., Bergmark, Å., Bäckman, O., Estrada, F., Fritzell, J., Lundberg, O., Sjöberg, O. and Szebehely, M. (2002) 'Welfare trends in Sweden: balancing the books for the 1990s', *Journal of European Social Policy*, vol 12, pp 329-46.

Palme, J., Bergmark, Å., Bäckman, O., Estrada, F., Fritzell, J., Lundberg, O., Sjöberg, O., Sommestad, L. and Szebehely, M. (2003) 'A welfare balance sheet for the 1990s. Final report of the Swedish Welfare Commission', *Scandinavian Journal of Public Health*, vol 31, Suppl 60.

Pampel, F.C. and Peters, E.H. (1995) 'The Easterlin effect', *Annual Review of Sociology*, vol 21, pp 163-94.

Parker, M., Ahacic, K. and Thorslund M. (2005) 'Health changes among Swedish oldest old: Prevalence rates from 1992 and 2002 show increasing health problems', *Journal of Gerontology: Medical Sciences*, vol 60A, pp 1351-5.

Pearce, N. and Davey Smith, G. (2003) 'Is social capital the key to inequalities in health?', *American Journal of Public Health*, vol 93, pp 122-9.

Phelan, J.C., Link, B.G., Diez-Roux, A., Kawachi, I. and Levin, B. (2004) 'Fundamental causes of social inequalities in mortality: a test of the theory', *Journal of Health and Social Behavior*, vol 45, pp 265-85.

Poortinga, W. (2006) 'Social capital: an individual or collective resource for health?', *Social Science and Medicine*, vol 62, pp 292-302.

Popay, J., Bartley, M. and Owen, C. (1993) 'Gender inequalities in health: social position, affective disorders and minor physical morbidity', *Social Science & Medicine*, vol 36, pp 21-32.

Popper, K. (1969) *Conjectures and refutations: The growth of scientific knowledge* (3rd edn), London: Routledge and Kegan Paul.

Poppius, E., Tenkanen, L., Hakama, M., Kalimo, R. and Pitkanen, T. (2003) 'The sense of coherence, occupation and all-cause mortality in the Helsinki Heart Study', *European Journal of Epidemiology*, vol 18, pp 389-93.

Portes, A. (1998) 'Social capital: its origins and application in modern sociology', *Annual Reviews of Sociology*, vol 24, pp 1-24.

Power, C., Manor, O. and Matthews, S. (1999) 'The duration and timing of exposure: effects of socioeconomic environment on adult health', *American Journal of Public Health*, vol 89, pp 1059-65.

Prestby, J., Wandersman, A. and Florin, F. (1990) 'Benefits, costs, incentive management and participation in voluntary organisations: a means to understanding and promoting empowerment', *American Journal of Community Psychology*, vol 18, pp 117-49.

Proposition (2002) *Mål för folkhälsan* [*Public health targets*], Government bill 2002/03:35, Stockholm: National Board of Health and Welfare.

Punnett, L. and Wegman, D.H. (2004) 'Work-related musculoskeletal disorders: the epidemiologic evidence and the debate', *Journal of Electromyography and Kinesiology*, vol 14, pp 13-23.

Punnett, L., Gold, J., Katz, J.N., Gore, R. and Wegman, D.H. (2004) 'Ergonomic stressors and upper extremity musculoskeletal disorders in automobile manufacturing: a one year follow up study', *Occupational and Environmental Medicine*, vol 61, pp 668-74.

Putnam R. (1993) *Making democracy work – Civic traditions in modern Italy*, Princeton, NJ: Princeton University Press.

Putnam, R. (2000) *Bowling alone: The collapse and revival of American community*, New York, NY: Simon and Schuster.

Rahkonen, O., Lahelma, E., Martikainen, P. and Silvertoinen, K. (2002) 'Determinants of health inequalities by income from the 1980s to the 1990s in Finland', *Journal of Epidemiology and Community Health*, vol 56, pp 442-3.

Rahkonen, O., Arber, S., Lahelma, E., Martikainen, P. and Silvertoinen, K. (2000) 'Understanding income inequalities in health among men and women in Britain and Finland', *International Journal of Health Services*, vol 30, pp 27-47.

Ray G.E., Cohen, R. and Secrist, M.E. (1995) 'Best friend networks of children across settings', *Child Study Journal*, vol 25, pp 169-88.

Riley III, J.L., Robinson, M.E., Wise, E.A., Myers, C.D. and Fillingim, R.B. (1998) 'Sex differences in the perception of noxious experimental stimuli: a meta-analysis', *Pain*, vol 74, pp 181-7.

Ringbäck Weitoft, G. and Rosén, M. (2005) 'Is perceived nervousness and anxiety a predictor of premature mortality and severe morbidity? A longitudinal follow up of the Swedish survey of living conditions', *Journal of Epidemiology and Community Health*, vol 59, pp 794-8.

Rodgers, G.B. (1979) 'Income and inequality as determinants of mortality: an international cross-section analysis', *Population Studies*, vol 33, pp 343-51 [reprinted in *International Journal of Epidemiology*, 2002, vol 31, pp 533-8].

Rognerud, M. and Zahl, P.-H. (2006) 'Social inequalities in mortality: changes in the relative importance of income, education and household size over a 27-year period', *European Journal of Public Health*, vol 16, pp 62-8.

Rose, R. (2000) 'How much does social capital add to individual health? A survey study of Russians', *Social Science and Medicine*, vol 51, pp 1421-35.

Rosén, M. and Haglund, B. (2005) 'From healthy survivors to sick survivors – implications for the twenty-first century', *Scandinavian Journal of Public Health*, vol 33, pp 151-5.

Rostila, M. (2004) 'Vart tog det "goda" arbetet vägen?' ['What happened to the "good" work?'], *Arbetsmarknad & Arbetsliv*, vol 10, pp 173-86.

Rothman, K.J. (2002) *Epidemiology: An introduction*, New York, NY: Oxford University Press.

Rothstein, B. (1998) *Just institutions matter: The moral and political logic of the universal welfare state*, Cambridge: Cambridge University Press.

Rothstein, B. (2001) 'Social capital in the social democratic welfare state', *Politics and Society*, vol 29, pp 207-41.

Rothstein, B. (2003a) 'Förtroende i det multikulturella samhället' ['Trust in the multicultural society'] in S. Holmberg and L. Weibull (eds), *Ju mer vi är tillsammans: tjugosju kapitel om politik, medier och samhälle: SOM-undersökningen 2003 [As long as we are together: Twenty-seven chapters about politics, mediums and society: The SOM-survey 2003]*, Göteborg: SOM-institutet, pp 75-81.

Rothstein, B. (2003b) *Sociala fällor och tillitens problem. [Social pitfalls and the problem with trust]*, Stockholm: SNS förlag.

Rothstein, B. and Kumlin, S. (2000) 'Demokrati, socialt kapital och förtroende' ['Democracy, social capital and trust'], in S. Holmberg and L. Weibull (eds) *Land, Du välsignade?: SOM-undersökningen 2000 [Land, thou blessed? The SOM-survey 2000]*, Göteborg: SOM-institutet, pp 49-62.

Rothstein, B. and Stolle, D. (2003) 'Social capital in Scandinavia', *Scandinavian Political Studies*, vol 26, pp 1-26.

Rowntree, S. (1901) *Poverty: A study of town life*, London: Macmillan.

Roxburgh, S. (1996) 'Gender differences in work and well-being: effects of exposure and vulnerability', *Journal of Health and Social Behavior*, vol 37, pp 265-77.

Rugulies, R. and Krause, N. (2005) 'Job strain, iso-strain, and the incidence of low back and neck injuries. A 7.5-year prospective study of San Francisco transit operators', *Social Science & Medicine*, vol 61, pp 27-39.

Runciman, W.G. (1966) *Relative deprivation and social justice*, London: Routledge and Kegan Paul.

Ryder, N.A. (1965) 'The cohort as a concept in the study of social change', *American Sociological Review*, vol 30, pp 843-61.

Ryff, C. and Singer, B. (1998) 'The contours of positive human health', *Psychological Inquiry*, vol 9, pp 1-28.

Ryland, E. and Greenfeld, S. (1991) 'Work stress and well being: an investigation of Antonovsky's sense of coherence model', *Journal of Social Behavior and Personality*, vol 6, pp 39-54.

Sagy, S., Antonovsky, A. and Adler, I. (1990) 'Explaining life satisfaction in later life: the sense of coherence model and activity theory', *Behavior, Health, and Aging*, vol 1, pp 11-25.

Samdahl, O. (1998) 'The school environment as a risk or resource for students' health-related behaviors and subjective well-being', Doctoral dissertation, Norway: Research Centre for Health Promotion, Faculty of Psychology, University of Bergen.

Savolainen, J., Suominen-Taipale, A.-L., Hausen, H., Harju, P., Uutela, A., Martelin, T. and Knuuttila, M. (2005) 'Sense of coherence as a determinant of the oral health-related quality of life: a national study in Finnish adults', *European Journal of Oral Sciences*, vol 113, pp 121-7.

Sayers, S.P., Jette, A.M., Haley, S.M., Heeren, T.C., Guralnik, J.M. and Fielding, R.A. (2004) 'Validation of the late-life function and disability instrument', *Journal American Geriatric Society*, vol 52, pp 1554-9.

Scheepers, P., Te Grotenhuis, M. and Gelissen, J. (2002) 'Welfare states and dimensions of social capital: cross-national comparisons of social contacts in European countries', *European Societies*, vol 4, pp 185-207.

Schnall, P.L., Landsbergis, P.A. and Baker, D. (1994) 'Job strain and cardiovascular disease', *Annual Review of Public Health*, vol 15, pp 381-411.

Schrijvers, C., van de Mheen, H., Stronks, K. and Mackenbach, J. (1998) 'Socioeconomic inequalities in health in the working population: the contribution of working conditions', *International Journal of Epidemiology*, vol 27, pp 1011-18.

Scott, J., Brynin, M. and Smith, R. (1995) 'Interviewing children in the British Household Panel Study', in J.J. Hox, B.F. van der Meulen, A.M. Janssens, L.T. Tavecchio and J.J.F. ter Laak (eds) *Advances in family research*, Amsterdam: Thesis Publishers, pp 259-66.

Sen, A. (1984) 'Poverty, relatively speaking', in A. Sen (ed) *Resources, values and development*, Cambridge, MA: Harvard University Press.

Sen, A. (1985a). 'Well-being, agency and freedom, the Dewey lectures 1984', *Journal of Philosophy*, vol 82, pp 169-221.

Sen, A. (1985b) *Commodities and capabilities*, Amsterdam: North Holland.

Sen, A. (1985c) 'A sociological approach to the measurement of poverty: a reply to professor Peter Townsend', *Oxford Economic Papers*, vol 37, pp 669-76.

Sen, A. (1987) *The standard of living: The Tanner lectures*, Cambridge: Cambridge University Press.

Sen, A. (1992) *Inequality re-examined*, Cambridge, MA: Harvard University Press.

Sen, A. (1995) 'Mortality as an indicator of economic success and failure', Innocenti Lectures, Inaugural lecture, Florence: UNICEF.

Sen, A. (2002) 'Why health equity?' *Health Economics*, vol 11, pp 659-66.

Shye, D., Mullooly, J.P, Freeborn, D.K. and Pope, C.R (1995) 'Gender differences in the relationship between social network support and mortality', *Social Science and Medicine*, vol 41, pp 935-47.

Sjostrom, H., Langius-Eklof, A. and Hjertberg, R. (2004) 'Well-being and sense of coherence during pregnancy', *Acta Obstetricia et Gynecologica Scandinavica*, vol 83, pp 1112-18.

Smith, P.M., Breslin, F.C. and Beaton, D.E. (2003) 'Questioning the stability of sense of coherence. The impact of socio-economic status and working conditions in the Canadian population', *Social Psychiatry and Psychiatric Epidemiology*, vol 38, pp 475-84.

Söderfeldt, M., Söderfeldt, B., Ohlsson, C.-G., Theorell, T. and Jones, I. (2000) 'The impact of sense of coherence and high-demand/low-control job environment on self-reported health, burnout and psychophysiological stress indicators', *Work & Stress*, vol 14, pp 1-15.

SOU Reports of the Government Commissions 2002:5 *Handlingsplan för ökad hälsa i arbetslivet* [*Action programme for improved health in working life*], Stockholm: Fritzes.

Sparén, P., Vågerö, D., Shestov, D.B., Plavinskaja, S. Parfenova, N., Hoptiar, V., Paturot, D. and Galanti, M.R. (2004) 'Long term mortality after severe starvation during the siege of Leningrad: prospective cohort study', *British Medical Journal*, vol 328, pp 11-20.

Spivack, G. and Marcus, J. (1987) 'Marks and classroom adjustment as early indicators of mental health at age twenty', *American Journal of Community Psychology*, vol 15, pp 35-55.

Ståhlberg, A.-C. (1994) 'Kvinnors ATP och avtalspensioner: Expertbilaga till pensionsarbetsgruppens betänkande' ['Women's supplementary pension, ATP and pension via collective agreements'] in *Report of the Government Commissions, SOU 1994:22 Bilaga B*. Stockholm: Fritzes.

Statistics Sweden (2002) *Livslängd, hälsa och sysselsättning* [*Life expectancy, health and employment*], Demographic reports 2002:3, Örebro: Statistics Sweden.

Statistics Sweden (2003) *Studie av bortfallet i 2000-års undersökningar av levnadsförhållanden (ULF). Bakgrundsfakta till befolknings- och välfärdsstatistik* [*Study of the non-response in the 2000's Surveys of Living Conditions (ULF) Background facts on the population and welfare statistics*], Report 2003:8, Stockholm: Statistics Sweden.

Statistics Sweden (2004) *Dödlighet efter utbildning, boende och civilstånd. Perioden 1986-2003* [*Mortality by education, type of housing and civil status. Period from 1986 to 2003*], Demographic reports 2004:4, Stockholm: Statistics Sweden.

Statistics Sweden (2005a) www.scb.se/templates/tableOrChart____25830.asp Stockholm: Statistics Sweden, updated 14 June 2006, accessed 7 February 2005.

Statistics Sweden (2005b) www.ssd.scb.se/databaser/makro/ Produkt.asp?produktid=AM0207, Stockholm: Statistics Sweden, updated 3 October 2006, accessed 29 August 2005.

Statistics Sweden (2005c) *Sysselsättning och arbetslöshet 1976-2004* [*Employment and unemployment 1976-2004*], Information från Arbetskraftsundersökningen 2005:1 [Information from the Labour Force Survey 2005:1], Stockholm: Statistics Sweden

Statistics Sweden and Swedish Work Environment Authority (2001) *Arbetsmiljöundersökningen 2001* [*Work Environment Survey 2001*], Stockholm: Statistics Sweden and Swedish Work Environment Authority.

Stolle, D. (2001) 'Getting to trust – an analysis of the importance of institutions, families, personal experiences and group membership', in P. Dekker and E.M. Uslaner (eds) *Social capital and participation in everyday life*, London: Routledge, pp 118-33.

Stouffer, S.A., Suchman, E.A., De Vinney, L.C., Star, S.A. and Williams, R.M. (1949) *The American soldier: Adjustment during army life*, vol 1, Princeton, NJ: Princeton University Press.

Stronks, K. van de Mheen, H.D. and Mackenbach, J.P. (1998) 'A higher prevalence of health problems in low income groups: does it reflect relative deprivation?', *Journal of Epidemiology and Community Health*, vol 52, pp 548-57.

Subramanian, S.V. and Kawachi, I. (2004) 'Income inequality and health: what have we learned so far?', *Epidemiologic Reviews*, vol 26, pp 78-91.

Subramanian, S.V., Kim, D.J. and Kawachi, I. (2002) 'Social trust and self-rated health in US communities: a multilevel analysis', *Journal of Urban Health*, vol 79, Suppl 1, pp 21-34.

Sundström, G. and Johansson, L. (2004) *Framtidens anhörigomsorg. Kommer de anhöriga vilja, kunna, orka ställa upp för de äldre i framtiden?* [*The future of informal care. Will and can informal carers provide care to older people in the future?*], Stockholm: National Board of Health and Welfare.

Suominen, S., Helenius, H., Blomberg, H., Uutela, A. and Koskenvuo, M. (2001) 'Sense of coherence as a predictor of subjective state of health: results of 4 years of follow-up of adults', *Journal of Psychosomatic Research*, vol 50, pp 77-86.

Surtees, P., Wainwright, N., Luben, R., Khaw, K.-T. and Day, N. (2003) 'Sense of coherence and mortality in men and women in the EPIC-Norfolk United Kingdom prospective cohort study', *American Journal of Epidemiology*, vol 158, pp 1202-9.

Svedberg, L. (2001) 'Spelar ideella och informella insatser någon roll för svensk välfärd?' ['Do non-profit and informal efforts play any role for the welfare of Sweden?'] in M. Szebehely (ed) *Välfärdstjänster i omvandling* [*Welfare services in transition*] Stockholm: Fritzes, pp 141-88.

SWEA (The Swedish Work Environment Authority) and Statistics Sweden (2001) *Negativ stress och ohälsa. Inverkan av höga krav, låg egenkontroll och bristande socialt stöd i arbetet,* [*Negative stress and ill-health. The effects of high demands, low control and lack of social support*] Report 2001:2, Stockholm: Statistics Sweden.

Swedish Integration Board (2003) *Rapport Integration 2003*, Norrköping: Integrationsverket.

Sweeting, H. (1995) 'Reversals of fortune? Sex differences in health in childhood and adolescence', *Social Science & Medicine*, vol 40, pp 77-90.

Sweeting, H. and West, P. (2003) 'Sex differences in health at ages 11, 13 and 15', *Social Science & Medicine*, vol 56, pp 31-9.

Szebehely, M. (1998) 'Changing divisions of carework: caring for children and frail elderly people in Sweden', in J. Lewis (ed) *Gender, social care and welfare restructuring in Europe*, Aldershot: Ashgate, pp 257-83.

Szebehely, M. (2000) 'Äldreomsorg i förändring' ['Transitions in the old age care system'], in M. Szebehely (ed) *Välfärd, vård och omsorg. SOU 2000:38* [*Government report 2000:38. Welfare and care*], Stockholm: Socialdepartementet.

Szebehely, M. (2005) 'Care as employment and welfare provision – child care and elder care in Sweden at the dawn of the 21st century', in H.M. Dahl and T.R. Eriksen (eds) *Dilemmas of care in the Nordic welfare state. Continuity and change*, Aldershot: Ashgate.

Tåhlin, M. (1987) 'Class mobility in a Swedish city', in E.J. Hansen, S. Ringen, H. Uusitalo and R. Erikson (eds) *Welfare trends in Scandinavian countries*, New York, NY: M.E. Sharpe, pp 181-213.

Tåhlin, M. (2001) 'Trettio års arbetsmiljösatsning – till vad nytta?' ['Thirty years of investments in work environment – what was the benefit?'] *Arbetsmarknad & Arbetsliv,* vol 7, pp 129-39.

Tak-Ying Shiu, A. (2004) 'Sense of coherence amongst Hong Kong Chinese adults with insulin-treated type 2 diabetes', *International Journal of Nursing Studies,* vol 41, pp 387-96.

Theorell, T. (2003) *Psykosocal miljö och stress* [*Psychosocial environment and stress*], Lund: Studentlitteratur.

Thorslund, M. and Lundberg, O. (1994) 'Health and inequalities among the oldest old', *Journal of Aging and Health*, vol 6, pp 51-69.

Thorslund, M., Lundberg, O. and Parker, M. (1993) 'Klass och ohälsa bland de allra äldsta. Studie visar allmängiltigt samband' ['Class and morbidity among the oldest old. A study shows a general connection'], *Läkartidningen*, vol 90, pp 3547-50, 3553.

Thorslund, M., Lennartsson, C., Parker, M.G. and Lundberg, O. (2004) 'De allra äldstas hälsa har blivit sämre' ['Health status of the oldest old has changed for the worse. Big differences between the sexes – health of women is worse than health of men as illuminated by new data'], *Läkartidningen*, vol 101, pp 1494-9.

Thoursie, A. (1998) *Studies on unemployment duration and on the gender wage gap*, Dissertation Series No 35, Stockholm: Swedish Institute for Social Research.

Titmuss, R.M. (1950) *Problems of social policy*, London: HMSO.

Titmuss, R.M. (1958) *Essays on the welfare state*, London: Allen & Unwin.

Tönnies, F. (1887/1957) *Community and society*, New York, NY: Harper Torchbooks.

Torpe, L. (2003) 'Social capital in Denmark: a deviant case?', *Scandinavian Political Studies*, vol 26, pp 27-48.

Torsheim, T. and Wold, B. (2001a) 'School-related stress, support, and subjective health complaints among early adolescents: a multilevel approach', *Journal of Adolescence*, vol 24, pp 701-13.

Torsheim, T. and Wold, B. (2001b) 'School-related stress, school support, and somatic complaints: a general population study', *Journal of Adolescent Research*, vol 16, pp 293-303.

Townsend, P. (1979) *Poverty in the United Kingdom*, Harmondsworth: Penguin.

Townsend, P. (1985) 'A sociological approach to the measurement of poverty – a rejoinder to professor Amartya Sen', *Oxford Economic Papers*, vol 37, pp 659-68.

Townsend, P. and Davidson, N. (1982) *Inequalities in health: The Black Report*, Harmondsworth: Penguin.

Trydegård, G.-B. (2000) 'From poorhouse overseer to production manager: one hundred years of old-age care in Sweden', *Ageing and Society*, vol 20, pp 571-98.

Turner, J.A. (1980) 'Computers in bank clerical functions: implications for productivity and the quality of life', Doctoral dissertation, Colombia University.

UNDP (United Nations Development Programme) (2004) *Human Development Report 2004: Cultural liberty in today's diverse world*, New York, NY: UN.

Uslaner, E. (2002) *The moral foundations of trust*, New York, NY: Cambridge University Press.

Vågerö, D. and Erikson, R. (1997) 'Socio-economic inequalities in morbidity and mortality in Western Europe', *Lancet*, vol 350, p 516.

Vågerö, D. and Illsley, R. (1995) 'Explaining health inequalities: beyond Black and Barker', *European Sociological Review*, vol 11, pp 219-41.

Vågerö, D. and Leon, D. (1994) 'Effect of social class in childhood and adulthood on adult mortality', *Lancet*, vol 343, pp 1224-5.

Vågerö, D. and Lundberg, O. (1989) 'Health inequalities in Britain and Sweden', *Lancet*, vol 334, pp 35-6.

Valkonen, T. (1989) 'Adult mortality and level of education: a comparison of six countries', in A.J. Fox (ed) *Health inequalities in European countries*, Aldershot: Gower.

Valkonen, T., Brancker, A., and Reijo, M. (1992) 'Mortality differentials between three populations – residents of Scandinavia, Scandinavian immigrants to Canada and Canadian-born residents of Canada, 1979-1985', *Health Report*, vol 4, pp 137-59.

Valkonen, T., Martikainen, P. and Blomgren, J. (2004) 'Increasing excess mortality among non-married elderly people in developed countries', *Demographic Research, Special Collection 2* (Article 12).

van den Heuvel, S.G., van der Beek, A.J., Blatter, B.M., Hoogendorn, W.E. and Bongers, P.M. (2005) 'Psychosocial work characteristics in relation to neck and upper limb symptoms', *Pain*, vol 114, pp 47-53.

van der Doef, M. and Maes, S. (1999) 'The job demand-control(-support) model and psychological well-being: a review of 20 years of empirical research', *Work & Stress*, vol 13, pp 87-114.

van Oorschot, W. and Arts, W. (2005) 'The social capital of European welfare states: the crowding out hypothesis revisited', *Journal of European Social Policy*, vol 15, pp 5-26.

Veenstra, G. (2000) 'Social capital, SES and health: an individual-level analysis', *Social Science & Medicine*, vol 50, pp 619-29.

Veenstra, G. (2005) 'Location, location, location: contextual and compositional health effects of social capital in British Columbia, Canada', *Social Science & Medicine*, vol 60, pp 2059-71.

Verbrugge, L.M. (1989) 'The twain meet: empirical explanations of sex differences in health and mortality', *Journal of Health and Social Behavior*, vol 30, pp 282-304.

Verbrugge, L.M. and Jette, A.M. (1994) 'The disablement process', *Social Science & Medicine*, vol 38, pp 1-14.

Vermeulen, M. and Mustard, C. (2000) 'Gender differences in job strain, social support at work, and psychological distress', *Journal of Occupational Health Psychology*, vol 5 pp 428-40.

Vingård, E., Alfredsson, L., Hagberg, M., Kilbom, Å., Theorell, T., Waldenström, M., Wigaeus Hjelm, E., Wiktorin, C., Hogstedt, C. and the MUSIC-Norrtälje Study Group (2000) 'To what extent do current and past physical and psychosocial occupational factors explain care-seeking for low back pain in a working population? Results from the Musculoskeletal Intervention Center-Norrtälje Study', *Spine*, vol 25, pp 493-500.

Volinn, E. and Punnett, L. (2001) 'Point of view', *Spine*, vol 26, pp 1902-3.

von Bothmer, M.I.K. and Fridlund, B. (2003) 'Self-rated health among university students in relation to sense of coherence and other personality traits', *Scandinavian Journal of Caring Sciences*, vol 17, pp 347-57.

Wagstaff, A. and van Doorslaer, E. (2000) 'Income inequality and health – what does the literature tell us?', *Annual Review of Public Health*, vol 21, pp 543-67.

Wahlstedt, K. (2001) 'Postal work – postal organizational changes as tools to improve health', Doctoral dissertation, Uppsala University.

Walters, V., McDonough, P. and Strohschein, L. (2002) 'The influence of work, household structure, and social, personal and material resources on gender differences in health: an analysis of the 1994 Canadian National Population Health Survey', *Social Science & Medicine*, vol 54, pp 677-92.

Watson, D. and Clark, L.A. (1984) 'Negative affectivity: the disposition to experience aversive emotional states', *Psychological Bulletin*, vol 96, pp 465-90.

West, P. (1997) 'Health inequality in the early years: is there equalisation in youth?', *Social Science & Medicine*, vol 44, pp 833-58.

West, P. and Sweeting, H. (2003) 'Fifteen, female and stressed: changing patterns of psychological distress over time', *Journal of Child Psychology and Psychiatry*, vol 44, pp 399-411.

West Pedersen, A. (2004) 'Inequality as relative deprivation. A sociological approach to inequality measurement', *Acta Sociologica*, vol 47, pp 31-49.

Wilkinson, R. (1992) 'Income distribution and life expectancy', *British Medical Journal*, vol 304, pp 165-8.

Wilkinson, R. (ed) (1986) *Class and health. Research and longitudinal data*, London: Tavistock.

Wilkinson, R.G. (1996) *Unhealthy societies: The afflictions of inequality*, London: Routledge.

Wolfe, A. (1989) *Whose keeper? Social science and moral obligation*, Berkeley, CA: University of California Press.

Wollebaek, D. and Selle, P. (2002) 'Does participation in voluntary associations contribute to social capital? The impact of intensity, scope, and type', *Nonprofit and Voluntary Sector Quarterly*, vol 31, pp 32-61.

Index

Page references for notes are followed by n

What works in tackling health inequalities?
Pathways, policies and practice through the lifecourse
Sheena Asthana and **Joyce Halliday**

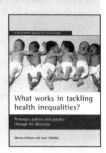

What works in tackling health inequalities?

Pathways, policies and practice through the lifecourse

Sheena Asthana and Joyce Halliday

"An authoritative and comprehensive account by two key researchers in this emerging and important new field." **Daniel Dorling**, Department of Geography, University of Sheffield

In recent years, tackling health inequalities has become a key policy objective in the UK. However, doubts remain about how best to translate broad policy recommendations into practice. This book identifies the key targets for intervention through a detailed exploration of the pathways and processes that give rise to health inequalities across the lifecourse. Authoritative yet accessible, the book provides a comprehensive account of theory, policy and practice.

Paperback £24.99 US$45.00 ISBN-13 978 1 86134 674 2
Hardback £65.00 US$119.95 ISBN-13 978 1 86134 675 9
240 x 172mm 624 pages March 2006
Studies in Poverty, Inequality and Social Exclusion series

Health inequalities
Lifecourse approaches
Edited by **George Davey Smith**

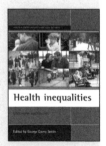

Health inequalities

Lifecourse approaches

Edited by George Davey Smith

"The good news for all his readers is that this warrior is armed with exceptional brains and great rhetorical gifts, and sees his task as 'the fearless description of how the world really is.'" **British Medical Journal**

"... a fascinating volume: provocative and challenging, often humorous but never dull." **Health Service Journal**

The lifecourse perspective on adult health and on health inequalities in particular, is one of the most important recent developments in epidemiology and public health. This book brings together, in a single volume, the work of one of the most distinguished academics in the field.

Paperback £25.00 US$39.95 ISBN-13 978 1 86134 322 2
240 x 172mm 608 pages August 2003
Studies in Poverty, Inequality and Social Exclusion series
INSPECTION COPY AVAILABLE

The political economy of health care
A clinical perspective
Julian Tudor Hart

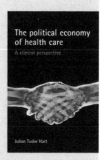

"Health care shaped by market forces and 'commodification' does not deliver services efficiently, let alone equitably. For those who support the principal of universal, equitable access to cost-effective health care, Julian Tudor Hart's radical vision of what is needed will come as a breath of inspiring fresh air." **Sir Iain Chalmers**, Editor, James Lind Library

This is a passionate analysis of the historical development, current state and potential future shape of the National Health Service by distinguished doctor and author, Julian Tudor Hart. Drawing on many years of clinical experience, Tudor Hart sets out to explore how the NHS might be reconstituted as a humane service for all (rather than a profitable one for the few) and a civilising influence on society as a whole.

Paperback £14.99 US$32.95 **ISBN-10** 1 86134 808 8; **ISBN-13** 978 1 86134 808 1

Hardback £55.00 US$69.95 **ISBN-10** 1 86134 809 6; **ISBN-13** 978 1 86134 809 8

234 x 156mm 336 pages April 2006

Health and Society series

To order copies of this publication or any other Policy Press titles please visit **www.policypress.org.uk** or contact:

In the UK and Europe:
Marston Book Services, PO Box 269, Abingdon, Oxon, OX14 4YN, UK
Tel: +44 (0)1235 465500
Fax: +44 (0)1235 465556
Email: direct.orders@marston.co.uk

In Australia and New Zealand:
DA Information Services, 648 Whitehorse Road Mitcham, Victoria 3132, Australia
Tel: +61 (3) 9210 7777
Fax: +61 (3) 9210 7788
E-mail: service@dadirect.com.au

In the USA and Canada:
ISBS, 920 NE 58th Street, Suite 300, Portland, OR 97213-3786, USA
Tel: +1 800 944 6190 (toll free)
Fax: +1 503 280 8832
Email: info@isbs.com